MW00888063

Praise
Yoga: The Secret

Danny Living is a devoted yogi and a genuinely nice, aware, and sensitive person. He has practiced yoga for many years and has great insight into what yoga is all about. I have posted "The Chemistry of Yoga" chapter from this book on my website under the Articles section; I think that it is brilliant. I heartily recommend, Danny's book, Yoga: The Secret, *and anything else that he may write.*

—David Williams, Senior Ashtanga Yoga Instructor
www.ashtangayogi.com

My favorite yoga teacher once shared that 'pain and suffering that has not yet occurred, needs to be avoided.' As all things have the potential to be manifest or unmanifest, the same is true for creating ease, health, and abundance. Yoga: The Secret *addresses this issue quite clearly and thoroughly. Instead of avoiding negative patterns, Danny Living suggests creating new, positive configurations as one performs a valuable activity for the body-mind, Ashtanga Yoga. Despite its associated discipline and intensity, I believe that Ashtanga Yoga provides space for the practitioner to explore affirmative life and thought patterns.* Yoga: The Secret *provides a map for the practitioner to find this place and to create nuances to help the space resonate uniquely.*

—Jim Vincenti, PhD, Portsmouth, NH

Yoga: The Secret *provides more than just crystal-clear instruction on the mechanics of Ashtanga Yoga. It also offers a roadmap for a healthy, positive outlook on life. As much for the mind and soul as it is for the body, this book is a must-read for anyone seeking more than a six-pack from their fitness routine.*

—Sal DeTraglia, Castilla-LaMancha (Spain)

Danny Living is the most positive person I know. In Yoga: The Secret, *Danny shows how he has used his personal yoga practice to heal his body, remove long-standing emotional blocks, and realize his wildest dreams.*

—J. Michael Parrish, Dean, San Jose State University

Yoga: The Secret

Yoga: The Secret

What you think matters

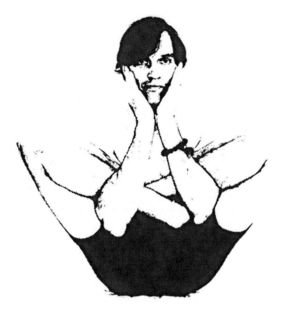

Danny Living

iUniverse, Inc.

New York Lincoln Shanghai

Yoga: The Secret
What you think matters

Copyright © 2007 by Danny Living

iUniverse books may be ordered through booksellers or by contacting:

iUniverse
2021 Pine Lake Road, Suite 100
Lincoln, NE 68512
www.iuniverse.com
1-800-Authors (1-800-288-4677)

Because of the dynamic nature of the Internet, any Web addresses or links contained in this book may have changed since publication and may no longer be valid.

CONSULT YOUR DOCTOR BEFORE BEGINNING THIS EXERCISE PROGRAM to reduce the risk of injury prior to attempting this or any other exercise program. Not all exercises are suitable for everyone and attempting this or any other program may result in injury. Any user of this exercise program assumes the risk of injury resulting from performing the exercises. The instructions and material contained herein are not intended to be a substitute for any medical advice. The author and distributors disclaim any liabilities or loss in connection with the use of the exercises or material herein.

ISBN: 978-0-595-44820-3 (pbk)
ISBN: 978-0-595-89137-5 (ebk)

Printed in the United States of America

Gratitude

I would like to dedicate this book to everyone who has ever watered my writing seed.

I am grateful to my beautiful wife, Kathy, whose abundant love and unwavering faith in me brought this book to you.

My children, Andy, Inge, Adam, and Stuart have inspired me to stretch beyond the limits I had placed upon myself (pun intended) and do what I love for the joy it brings. They remind me of the Native American saying, "We don't inherit the Earth from our ancestors, we borrow it from our children."

I am deeply grateful to the many people who have encouraged me along the way, particularly:

- *Phil Kennedy, who helped guide me to the wellspring of self-love, forgiveness and healing that waited patiently inside me.*
- *Dr. Joe Vitale, whose inspiration helped me find the gold in my life.*
- *David Williams the most heavy-duty yogi on the planet. David: You have been my Tat Wala Baba.*
- *Mrs. Winnings, my fourth grade teacher, the kind soul who told a ten-year old little boy that did not think very much of himself that he was smart and a good writer.*

Mrs. Winnings, wherever you are now, thank you!

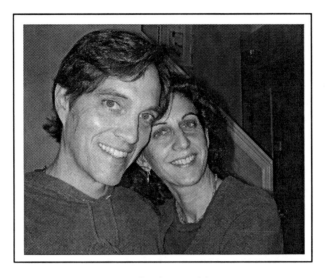

It was the love of love,
the love that swallows up all else,
a grateful love,
a love of nature, of people,
of animals,
a love engendering
gentleness and goodness
that moved me
and that I saw in you.

—William Carlos Williams

"The gold in a person's life is in the area where they're afraid ..."
—JOE VITALE

"The best way to become acquainted with a subject is to write a book about it."
—BENJAMIN DISRAELI

"The paper, ink, and other material in this book may not be worth the money you pay for it; but if the ideas suggested by it bring you thousands of dollars, you have not been wronged by those who sold it to you; they have given you a great use value for a small cash value."
—WALLACE WATTLES, *The Science of Getting Rich*

Contents

Chapter 1

How the Law of Attraction Got This Book to You

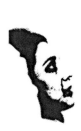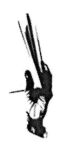

Get rid of the idea that God wants you to sacrifice yourself for others, and that you can secure his favor by doing so; God requires nothing of the kind.
What he wants is that you should make the most of yourself, for yourself, and for others; and you can help others more by making the most of yourself than in any other way.
—WALLACE WATTLES, The Science of Getting Rich

All of us tend to put off living. We are all dreaming of some magical rose garden over the horizon—instead of enjoying the roses that are blooming outside our windows today.
—DALE CARNEGIE

Go confidently in the direction of your dreams! Live the life you've imagined. As you simplify your life, the laws of the universe will be simpler.
—HENRY DAVID THOREAU

I wrote this book in 30 days.

The last chapter in the book is more or less a letter I wrote to David Williams, one of the most senior Ashtanga Yoga practitioners in the world. It was my intention to send him a copy when the book was published.

A week after I finished the first draft of the book, I wrote a simple sentence on a note card that I stuck to my bathroom mirror.

I looked at it every day. The note card said:

> *Someday David Williams is going to call me and I am going to go to Maui.*

I don't know where the idea to do that came from, but I trusted it.

Then, a few months later, my whole life turned upside down. I left a failing marriage, deciding that alone was better than modeling a poor marriage to my children. My ex-wife thought all I needed was a little R&R, so she suggested I take the kids somewhere nice, like Jamaica.

Well, there was no way of getting last-minute passports for the kids, so the travel agent suggested Hawaii (as my criterion was beaches and no passports for kids and no Florida, which we had gone to many times for the previous 10 years). There was no reasonable accomodations anywhere in Hawaii at the last minute. A day later, the travel agent called and said she'd found a place in Maui that a person was renting for $100 a night. She sent me some pictures.

I looked at the pictures: You could spit in the ocean (with a healthy neck snap) from the balcony. So, I booked it.

All of a sudden, I remembered my note card, which was now in my apartment in a drawer and on a whim, I emailed David Williams and told him I would be in Maui the next week and asked if I could meet him.

I still remember how shocked and surprised I was when he called the next day.

Three days later, I was in his garage, doing yoga.

Unreal.

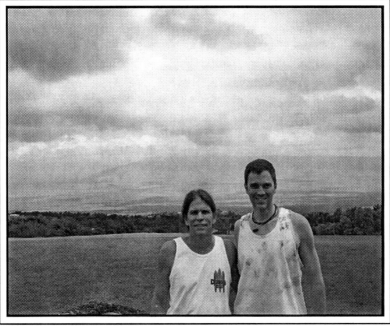

Senior Ashtanga Yoga Instructor David Williams and me in Maui, 2004

So, how did I write the book in 30 days?

Once I made up my mind that I was going to write the book, it literally poured out of me. I sometimes felt like someone else was doing the writing and I was just doing my best to type and keep up. Do the math: take the number of pages in this book, divide by 30 and you get a number of pages a day. 30 days later and there, you have it.

A few months after meeting David Williams, a person I knew set up a makeshift studio in his living room and for the next two hours he took a couple hundred pictures, two pictures of each pose. In some of the pictures, you could see my hands brushing the ceiling.

I had a friend crop the pictures when I had them on on a picture CD and I put them in the book …

Then the book sat.

I felt at times like I had given birth to a baby then locked it in a room.

I had set an intention of sharing my story with the world when it was finished, but once the book was finished, I was too scared to put myself out there.

I printed out a copy and sent it to David. He called when he got it and he asked me when I was going to publish it.

I froze. I said as soon as I found a publisher. He said "Alright" and said to send him a copy.

Whenever I would imagine taking the next step, which was trying to publish the book, I would always feel afraid. I am not sure if I was afraid of putting a book out there with pictures of me mostly naked that scared me. I don't know if the fact that the book contained personal details about me that made me feel vulnerable.

When I finished the book, I remember feeling exhilarated and thinking I wanted everyone in the world to read it.

Really.

But the more I thought about it, the more afraid I became.

There it sat. Done. Finished. Ready.

There I sat, frozen.

For three years.

Then, a funny thing happened. Someone brought the movie *The Secret* to our house and we watched it. Then, my wife and I bought it. She said, "Let's watch it for 30 days and see what happens to us."

So, we began watching *The Secret* every day.

About a week later, Kathy and I were practicing yoga with our friend Karen. I had emailed her a chapter of my book that had some practice tips.

That morning after practice, I asked her if she had read the excerpt.

She said she had and said, "Can I ask you a question? Why haven't you published this?"

That was the million-dollar question I had been asking myself.

I told her the truth. I told her I was afraid.

"Of what? It's good book. You're a good writer," she assured me.

I told her some of my reasons for feeling afraid. They sounded lame.

I tried to give her a concrete excuse. I told her that I wanted to re-shoot the pictures to add in variations and that I was looking for a photographer. Kathy and I talked about it and I had an inspired thought: Take the pictures in the place where you feel the most loved.

Home.

Ask and you shall receive. Great.

The Universe was going to see this book published no matter how much I protested.

When I looked at the original pictures, in addition to the imperfections, like seeing my hands touching the ceiling in the house where the pictures where shot, I looked scared and sad. I decided I would re-shoot the pictures. Since the original pictures were taken, I had become a raw foodist. I also had healed many old hurts, except for part of me that was afraid to publish my book. But, inside and out, I felt much healthier.

If I was going to go all the way and publish this book, I decided I wanted to look happy in the pictures. I wanted the pictures to reflect how I felt on the inside.

At the time the original pictures were taken, I could bend myself into most of the poses. But, yoga is more about what you feel on the inside then how you look on the outside. The original camera work captured more than my body. My emotion was there too.

So, we re-shot the pictures in my home with Kathy right there with me.

I guess I wanted everyone to see a happy Danny Living.

Things began to happen.

A week after my conversation with Karen and in week two of watching *The Secret*, Kathy and I were driving to the city, listening to a recording of a conversation between Dr. Joe Vitale and Bill Harris, two of the stars of the movie, *The Secret*. Bill Harris was asking Joe about Joe's book *The Attractor Factor*. Joe said that he'd been afraid to publish the book originally because it contained a lot of personal information. But, he was finally convinced to publish the book and it ended up being the work that he was most proud of and his best seller.

Joe said he wrote the book to share with his sister, but never intended it to go beyond there. When he finally published it, it was his most successful book … I think *because* it showed his vulnerability. People could connect with it. I have read some of Joe's books and I think it is his best work.

He said on the program:

"The gold in a person's life is in the area where they're afraid …"

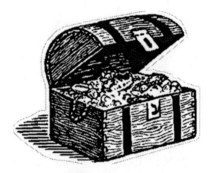

When he said that, Kathy poked me with a friendly elbow, "You're supposed to publish your book, Babes," she said.

"What book?" I asked. I knew exactly what book.

"Your yoga book …"

Oh, *that* book.

So, I took a deep breath. The next day, I emailed Joe and asked for his help. I included a short version of my story and sent him a chapter.

The next day, I got a wonderful email from his personal assistant, telling me that, while Joe was too busy to read my book because of an increased demand for appearances resulting from the success of the movie *The Secret*, she was happy to give me some resources.

I hooked up with a firm that sends a query letter to emails of legitimate agents and publishers. They helped me create a great letter, and they sent it out on my behalf. The next morning, the positive responses from publishers and agents started rolling in like high tide.

A couple days later, I dared to start imagining some of the publicity I would need to generate to get the book out to the masses, and acting on an inspired thought, I Googled "book publicists" and started skimming through websites. I was attracted to one name in particular, selected the *Contact Us* button and filled out a short form. I shoveled in the content of my query letter and left my email and home phone.

15 minutes later, the phone rang. It was the publicist I had just written. As in *Contact Us*.

She was interested in publicizing *my* book … I told her my story and it turns out she knows …

Joe Vitale.

She told me to self-publish the book and told me to call her when it was in print.

Whoa.

She asked about the state of the book. I told her I wanted to re-shoot the pictures. She said, "How soon can you be done?" I told her I would commit to having the pictures finalized and dumped into the book within two weeks.

She also gave me the name of a guy on the east coast that helps authors market their material. She told me, coincidentally, that she'd just spoken to him that morning. I called him later that afternoon and he gave me some more resources to self-publish, getting an ISBN number, the right book size, format, etc. He offered to help with press releases and mentioned his media contacts. It turns out that he is a yogi and, a friend of …

Joe Vitale.

Joe Vitale was becoming my Kevin Bacon.

I checked out the guy on the east coast's website and he had endorsements from Jack "Chicken Soup for the Soul" Canfield as well as many other famous authors for his marketing genius.

I unfroze.

I let the baby out to play, grow, and meet the world.

I am very grateful for all this, to say the least, especially all the encouragement.

My fourth grade teacher, Mrs. Winings, who I mention in the book, told me I was smart and a good writer.

Kathy, my kids, David Williams and so many others (and you all know who you are) have encouraged me along the way. No matter what happens to me as my life unfolds, I know that I am already the richest man I know!

As David Williams says, "yoga is for every body. Whether you 9 or 99."

A friend of mine read an excerpt of this book and told me that it was more than a book about yoga.

Read on.

Chapter 2

The Car Accident That Got Me to Try Yoga

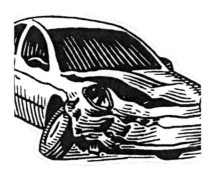

It is important to expect nothing, to take every experience, including the negative ones, as merely steps on the path, and to proceed.
—RAM DAS

The guru is the one who lights your candle, the one who flicks your switch.
—DAVID WILLIAMS

My first introduction to yoga came in the form of a Christmas gift.

One Christmas, I found myself holding a small, lightweight package in my hands. As everyone else tore into his or her gifts, I slowly opened mine. I found myself looking at three *Bryan Kest Power yoga* tapes. Not one. Three.

Yoga.

I was speechless. Have you ever had to open a gift and pretend to look happy and surprised?

I looked up. I arranged my face into Happy and Surprised. The slight smile. Eyebrows up. Anna, the person who had given me the gift was looking at me expectantly. I smiled, holding the tapes.

"What did you get?" someone else asked.

"Yoga tapes," I said, trying to hold that smile. I held the tapes up for everyone to see. I brought the tapes back down into my lap quickly and looked down at the picture on the cover of the first tape.

A bare-chested man with dark with shoulder-length hair held both arms straight overhead, hands clasped and index fingers steepled. He was standing, bowed slightly to one side, looking upward. A lot of hair was visible under his armpits.

Sorry, Bryan.

Yoga?

I held the tapes and the torn wrapping paper in my hands. Before I could set the tapes to the side, Anna was seated next to me talking excitedly.

Uh, oh.

"Okay," she began. "I want you to try this. I heard you liked to exercise. I studied with Bryan for several years and I think you're really going to like yoga."

She continued, "Watch the first tape all the way through, then rewind it and try it. If you don't like it …" She shrugged. "Then, at least you can say you tried it. Promise me you'll at least try it."

I promised to try it, but I confess I was skeptical to say the least.

Several years earlier, a mini-van going 45 mph had rear-ended me. I was sitting in my car at a stoplight. The driver had been talking on a cell phone and never even braked according to one witness. The police confirmed there were no skid marks. One minute I was waiting for the light to change and in the next instant, my car was crashing into the car in front of me. The impact launched me out of my seat and my chest hit the steering wheel, and my knees banged into the bottom of the dashboard. My neck snapped forward and back. I thought I was okay at first. Then, I started to feel sick to my stomach. When I sat down on the curb next to my crushed car, my neck and back started to hurt. An ambulance took me from the scene of the accident to the local emergency room. I am grateful that the car I drove at the time was a 1986 Ford Crown Victoria. All that extra metal probably saved me from a worser fate. The impact left me with a constant low back pain and stiffness in my neck that never really went away.

For the next two years, I lived in almost constant pain. I missed a month of work and had to take a powerful anti-inflamatory pain relievers just to make it through the day. The pain would get so bad that I would start to perspire an hour before my next dosage. I developed insomnia. The pain would wake me up from a sound sleep and I would get up in the middle of the night and walk my dog to town a few miles away or go downstairs and lay on the couch and watch TV until it was time to go to work.

It was a nightmare.

I had been active since I was a teenager. I had been a long-distance runner, a martial artist and loved to exercise. After the accident, I really could not do much of anything without hurting.

Pain is a funny thing. I didn't know what I know now, so the idea that I'd attracted the accident and that I was attracting more pain by focusing so much of my attention on it was nowhere within my awareness.

I only knew that I hurt all the time. The pain coupled with the lack of sleep caused me to sink into a depression that eventually left me with the feeling of moving through each day in a detached fog.

The idea that yoga would change any of that was not even a possibility that I was remotely considering. The only reason I was going to watch the tape and try it was because I said I would.

But my heart was not really in it.

So, on December 26th, 2000, I watched the tape as instructed, rewound it, and then tried to follow along.

I would like to report to you that I was gracefully able to manage the poses presented by Bryan Kest and demonstrated by his class of whom I now know to be accomplished yoga practitioners, including Bryan's brother Jonny and Sean Corn.

While I followed the tape, I was very aware of two things: my stiff lower and my lack of enthusiasm. At the halfway point, I was already dreading the next time I saw Anna and mentally rehearsing my heartfelt speech in which I'd sadly shake my head from side to side and say, No, I won't be doing any more yoga.

At the end of the tape, Bryan had the students in the class lie on their backs with their eyes closed, feet slightly apart and relaxed, arms at their sides, palms facing up. This relaxing music played and coupled with his soothing voice, I must have fallen asleep.

The next thing I knew, I heard the "click" of the machine stopping and the whirring of the tape rewinding. I felt like I'd awoken from the most restful sleep I'd had since I was a child. And the pain was gone. Wait. My back didn't hurt.

I slowly sat up and within ten minutes, the slow, dull ache came back.

But for those wonderful ten minutes, I felt good.

The next day, I did the whole tape again, thinking that if I skipped a single step, I wouldn't get the same result.

I was hooked.

After a month, I stopped taking pain relievers. I started to sleep more. I started to feel good more often.

I think, in retrospect, the guided relaxation at the end of the tape and the lingering peaceful feeling was what drew me back to yoga practice each day. I discovered just how much I *needed* yoga.

Anna's gift arrived right when I was ready to receive it.

Anna was my first teacher. Bryan Kest was my second teacher.

No one was more surprised than me.

Discovering Ashtanga Yoga

After making my way through all three tapes, I became interested in the yoga *behind* Power yoga. I visited Bryan Kest's website and read his biography. I learned that Bryan had studied with David Williams. The biography mentioned that David Williams had learned from someone named Pattabhi Jois. And, I learned the yoga behind the yoga was called *Ashtanga Yoga*.

So, I got a hold of an Ashtanga Yoga tape and for the next year or so, I followed along with the soft-spoken voice and graceful practice of Richard Freeman.

Richard Freeman was my next teacher.

In addition, I read all I could find about Ashtanga Yoga on the internet, on message boards, the many Ashtanga web sites, hungrily drinking up anything I could find on the subject.

Soon, I had many teachers.

Chapter 3

Finding My Yoga Teacher

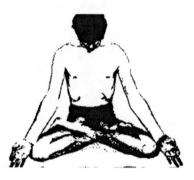

Teachers open the door. You enter by yourself.
—CHINESE PROVERB

When the five senses and the mind are still, and the reasoning intellect rests in silence, then begins the highest path. This calm steadiness of the senses is called yoga. Then one should become watchful, because yoga comes and goes.
—KATHA UPANISHAD

Okay, so where do you find *your* yoga teacher?

Know this first: I believe that yoga is a gift. Anyone that gives the gift of yoga to *someone willing to learn and ready to receive it* is a yoga teacher.

The greatest teachers use love and words of encouragement as the real tools of their trade.

The teacher provides the love and encouragement and offers from their experiences through some form of physical, verbal or written expression.

What happens in the mind and the body of the student *after* the teacher's love, encouragement and expressions is mostly up to the student.

I know firsthand what a difference a teacher's love and words of encouragement makes in the life of a student.

There is nothing like it.

Yet I still have had no *official* yoga teacher.

Much of my yoga practice has been a solitary, internal journey.

This means that much of the love and encouragement I have received has come from within.

I have discovered *within myself* the greatest yoga teacher.

Chapter 4

Meeting the Yoga Dancer

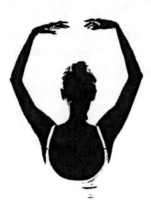

Hide not your talents, they for use were made.
What's a sun-dial in the shade?
—BENJAMIN FRANKLIN

One of my favorite internet sites is www.yogadancer.com. The site includes an index of asanas (yoga poses) listed alphabetically by their Sanskrit name. Go to the site and select the index. The index contains all the letters of the alphabet, each underlined to indicate a hyperlink. When you click on any letter of the alphabet in the index, you "jump" to a two-column table with all the asanas that begin with that letter of the alphabet. The table's left column has the Sanskrit name of the asana. The right column has the English translation or description.

For example, click on **S** and you "jump" to the "S" asanas like:

Samasthitih	Standing or Mountain Pose

Many of the indexed asanas have pictures of yogis (male) and yoginis (female) demonstrating each asana and its variations. Occasionally, you may find some instructions. Finding these step-by-step instructions is like finding little nuggets of gold if you are struggling with an asana, lack a teacher, or simply want to read someone else's tips.

The site is also a helpful aid when trying to decipher Sanskrit-rich technical descriptions and instructions for performing asanas. If you are not familiar with yoga's Sanskrit terminology, these technical instructions for asanas can be difficult to read and understand.

The indexed table of asanas became my "pocket" travel dictionary and a virtual "teacher" to guide me through the land of yoga.

An Ashtanga Yogini I only know as Christine maintains www.yogadancer.com. The site has an open invitation to visitors to contribute, whether it be photos, indentifying an unknown person in a picture demonstrating an asana, links to other related material, or instructions.

One day while looking at her site, I felt inspired to write her. Beyond the physical layout of the site, the links and the pictures, I suddenly imagined a person who so loved yoga that they decided to create a site for others as a small expression of gratitude—a way to give back.

While I did plenty of "taking" from the site, I had never contributed. However, my travels throughout the rest of the internet in search of yoga material had brought me in contact with other pictures and descriptions that I knew to be "gaps" in Christine's site, asanas without photos, etc.

Though I noted the gaps in her site, I never took the time to share or contribute anything.

So, on a whim, I emailed Christine. I had known for some time there was no photo or instructions for Nauli on her site (Nauli is a yogic exercise that involves blowing all your air out, sucking in your stomarch, puffing out your ribs cage and "churning" your stomach to massage your internal organs—for more information on Nauli, go to the table of contents and refer to the chapter in this book on Nauli called *Learning the Freaky Stomach Exercise*). I had found a good description of Nauli (with explanatory text *and* demonstration photos) on another website. I sent her the link.

Almost as an afterthought, I decided to include a little note of thanks and *encouragement*. So, I included in the email that I found her website to be a priceless resource, saying in particular that I really appreciated when an asana on her site included step-by-step instructions, like modification asanas/photos leading up to the final form of an asana. I had learned Padmasana (the Lotus Posture) using her site.

You never know when your words of encouragement can change the course of someone's life.

The next day, I got her reply. In it, she thanked me for the feed-back. She also mentioned she was working on one particular asana at the time. I *thought* she meant that she needed "instructions" for *her own* practice. Later, I learned she was only trying to find writ-ten instructions and/or step-by-step modification asanas leading up to the final form of the asana to *post* on her site *for others*. It turns out Christine is an instructor at an Ashtanga Yoga center.

In my ignorant determination to "help" the person who had helped me, I brushed off my technical writing skills and wrote detailed step-by-step instructions for the asana in question. I had managed to contort myself into this asana a year before and now could do it easily. I really believed I could describe the "how to" in enough detail, including internal and alignment tips, that *my writ-ten words alone* could "teach" her the asana. I sent her my instruc-tions.

The next day, there was another reply in my inbox.

She said she really liked my instructions and asked my permis-sion to *use them on her website*! She said that while she received plenty of photo submissions, detailed written instructions like mine were rare.

At the end of her message, she wrote:

If I could be so presumptuous, I would love it if you felt like narrating your practice. You do write well. Unlike most Ashtangis, particularly self-taught ones, you speak other yoga languages in your descriptions.

Chapter 5

Watering the Writing Seed

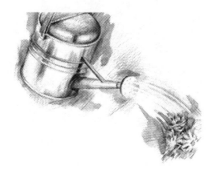

Let us be grateful to people who make us happy; they are the charming gardeners who make our souls blossom.
—MARCEL PROUST

An understanding heart is everything in a teacher, and cannot be esteemed highly enough. One looks back with appreciation to the brilliant teachers, but with gratitude to those who touched our human feeling. The curriculum is so much necessary raw material, but warmth is the vital element for the growing plant and for the soul of the child.
—CARL JUNG

A teacher effects eternity;
he can never tell where his influence stops.
—HENRY ADAMS

We know what we are, but know not what we may be.
—WILLIAM SHAKESPEARE, *Hamlet*

Her reply suddenly brought back memories of my fourth grade teacher.

I remembered the day my teacher, Mrs. Winings (pronounced WHY-NINGS), read a letter I wrote aloud to the rest of the class. One of the other teachers was sick, and Mrs. Winings had taken it upon herself to task each student in the class with writing Miss Janowski a "get well" letter. I didn't really know much about Miss Janowski, so I tried to think of as many nice things to say about her as I could to encourage her and make her feel better.

Mrs. Winings told me after class that I was one of the best writers in the whole school and that I had a "gift" for writing.

Ironically, my career as a writer began with *her* words of encouragement about *my* words of encouragement.

Those words of encouragement changed my life.

"I'm afraid that novel in you will have to come out"

I continued writing in high school and college, writing short stories and poetry, often receiving praise and encouragement from my teachers.

For a number of years, I made my living as a technical writer. Later, I discovered email. Email was a great way to keep in touch with people, share my thoughts, or offer encouragement. Email became my primary outlet for my "gift" for writing.

Over the years, people occasionally have said to me, "You're *really* a good writer, you should write a book."

And in my mind I always thought, "Yeah, but a book *about what*?"

All these years later, with a real passion for yoga and an invitation to narrate my practice, I suddenly found my book's *about what*.

A person I worked with years ago gave me a cartoon of a man sitting in a doctor's office in his underwear. A doctor is talking to the man. The caption reads, "I'm afraid that novel in you will have to come out."

The person who gave me the cartoon had written the words **Danny** at the beginning of the doctor's diagnosis.

The person who gave the cartoon to me is an accomplished writer named Jeff. At the time, Jeff wrote articles for a racing magazine. The company where we both worked often enlisted Jeff's help to write and edit the company's annual report. He also contributed to a variety of company publications in which the help of an expert writer was needed. The president of the company called him personally.

Jeff was one of the people who told me I had a talent for writing. I still have the cartoon, Jeff.

Truthfully, I suspect that I was born with the same "ability" or "talent' for writing that is in each one of us. I think all those people who encouraged my writing were not really just encouraging my writing. They were encouraging me.

I am a better person because of each of them and their words of encouragement.

Not knowing any better, I believed each and every one of them.

I think abilities are just another word for gifts or talents. If I can use a gardening analogy, I think that gifts or talents are like seeds. I like to think that when we are born, people are given many of the same gifts or talents or seeds.

But, not all seeds get watered.

My Favorite Teacher

Back on that day in fourth grade, I believe Mrs. Winings was the first person to water my "writing" seed.

She was my favorite teacher. Mrs. Winings used to read books out loud to us, using different voices for all the different characters in the stories. She taught us, through her own apparent love of reading, to love reading ourselves. I can close my eyes today and still see her sitting behind her old wooden desk, looking down at a book in her hands (*The Secret Garden, Pollyanna*), with her glasses halfway down her nose. Sometimes, the whole afternoon was dedicated to reading and our other books stayed inside our desks. No one complained. Those were magical afternoons.

I can still hear her voice, with its unique Southern twang.

Even though she was well past retirement age at the time, she still taught school because she clearly loved to teach. I doubt she was doing it for the money being that my parish was a poor one. A child soon knows which teachers love to teach and which are just doing it for the money. I could just tell by the enthusiasm she put into each class that she loved what she was doing.

Mrs. Winings often told us about her childhood on a farm. I remember a story she shared with us about the time her family's favorite cow died. She told us everyone in her family stood over the cow's body and cried, *including* her father.

One day Mrs. Winings slipped and fell on the ice in front of school while we were all lined up to come in from recess. We all laughed. One of the other teachers immediately yelled at us for laughing, shouting, "You should all be ashamed of yourselves!" Mrs. Winings picked herself up and began to laugh. Then, in a kind voice, she gently scolded the other teacher for yelling at us, saying that seeing an old woman slip and fall *was* funny.

She was wonderful.

Mrs. Winings always told me how smart I was. She put me in her advanced classes. Being in the advanced classes meant that you were taught in a separate classroom and given different books and material that was supposed to be more challenging.

Having someone like her tell me that I was good at writing *and* smart made a part of me feel 10-feet tall.

As a self-conscious fourth grader who was not very good at sports, having someone important to me say that I was good at something *and* smart filled me with just enough self-esteem to help me survive childhood. No matter what happened to me on the playground, or what the other kids said, or how often I was picked last for teams, or how often I felt lonely, none of that could take away the fact that Mrs. Winings said I was smart and a good writer.

The memory of that day in class when Mrs. Wining told me that I was a good writer and how I would feel when she would tell me how smart I was has served as a great lesson to me. I try to remember to encourage and compliment others whenever I can.

You never know when you are going to be a Mrs. Winings to someone.

Mrs. Winings, wherever you are, the hug you gave me on the last day of school—as I hid behind my mom and told you that you were my favorite teacher—has returned to you.

This book is my gift to the yoga community … my way to give back.

I would like to dedicate it to everyone who has ever watered my writing seed.

Chapter 6

Why Do I Have to Bend Myself Like a Pretzel?

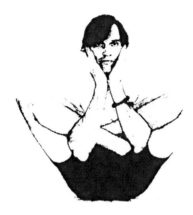

Though we travel the world over to find the beautiful, we must carry it with us or we find it not.
—RALPH WALDO EMERSON

So why do yoga practitioners bend themselves into all those pretzel-like poses?

I think the better question is this:

What are they looking for?

Asanas are a Map to the Body's Secret Hiding Places

Asanas provide us with a map to the body's secret hiding places for tension and reveal the logical channels with which joy flows through the body when unobstructed.

25

You are the explorer, the treasure hunter, traveling the body each time you practice in search of tension, guided by the asanas. When you discover tension in the body, be happy for you are finding the key to a buried treasure!

Each time you discover, release and resolve tension, you are rewarded with the good "feeling" that accompanies the release of joy that is now able to travel freely through the unobstructed channel. The "feeling" is both pleasant and *addictive*, inspiring and encouraging you to continue your daily journey in search of more tension.

Every victory over tension, through the discovery and resolution of *what has caused the tension in the first place,* brings with it a feeling of peace and contentment. This creates a wonderful economy in which *effort* results in a *reward*. The cycle of effort and reward becomes the cornerstone of practice.

The way you learn asanas varies by your circumstances, access to teachers, other yoga students and resource material.

Believe that your learning is *only* limited by the amount of time you are willing to dedicate to learning yoga, your thirst for knowledge, your commitment to *regular* practice and how much you allow yoga to permeate *the rest* of each day *after practice*.

If you listen to your body, each time you practice you will learn something. Each asana offers to teach you something about yourself and something about the asana.

Eventually the asanas are of secondary concern and the focus becomes the release of tension, the breath, and allowing joy to flow freely throughout the body.

You come to appreciate that this joy changes your thoughts, ultimately changing how you see the world and relate to the people around you.

I believe the primary purpose of asanas is to help us find tension in our body, discover its cause and release it.

When tension is released, channels within the body become unblocked and joy flows unobstructed.

Chapter 7

Imagine Your Body is a House

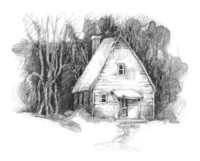

Unexpressed emotion is stored in the muscles of the body.
—WILHELM REICH

The sorrow which has no vent in tears may make other organs weep.
—HENRY MAUDSLEY

Over the years, your bodies become walking autobiographies, telling friends and strangers alike of the minor and major stresses of your lives.
—MARILYN FERGUSON

A bodily disease which we look upon as whole and entire within itself, may, after all, be but a symptom of some ailment in the spiritual part.
—NATHANIEL HAWTHORNE

Imagine your body is a large home with a series of rooms. Imagine that your body "house" has hidden within it some rooms filled with clutter and stale air, as they have been closed off for some time. Each of *these* rooms represents an area of the body where tension has been stored behind a sticky door.

The sticky door represents the tension itself and the contents of the room, the tension's cause.

Each asana will lead you to a room. Do you feel tension in an asana? What's *behind* the tension? What's *inside* the room with the sticky door?

In Ashtanga Yoga, the asanas become progressively more challenging as you move through the asanas in each series. Each asana prepares you for the next asana. Each asana series prepares us for the next asana series. Each series of asanas serves to open a logical group of "rooms" in your house. Every asana and series of asanas offers opportunities to release tension and open channels within the body.

And release joy.

But how does the tension get in the body in the first place? How does releasing tension release joy?

And if releasing tension releases joy, how are the two connected?

The Tension/Joy Connection

Joy is a term to describe a "feeling." Joy is a physical manifestation of love.

Tension is a term to describe a "feeling." Tension is a physical manifestation of fear.

The opposite of love isn't hate. It's fear.

When joy is released, it fills you with positive *feelings* that generate positive thoughts. Positive thoughts *help* give you a positive view of your past, present, and future worlds, ultimately changing the way you relate to the people in those worlds.

With this "new" worldview and way of relating to people, you create joy instead of tension.

Patiently practice the asanas repeatedly. Take deep, full inhales and exhales, and press *gently* without crossing the threshold of pain into the areas of discovered tension, asking, "What has caused this tension?" By doing so, you are pushing tenderly against each sticky door, not forcibly, until the door opens.

- When you are tense, you tend to *hold* your breath, or breathe more shallowly.
- When you are relaxed, you naturally *release* the breath, and breathe more deeply.

Consciously breathing deeply brings your attention to the connection between your breath and any associated physical responses in the body. During your practice, you are *training your body to relax* by providing one of the fundamental physical companions of relaxation: deep full breaths.

Go back to the house. Within each room, if you are patient, you will eventually discover the source of the tension: someone you need to forgive, grief, sadness, frustration, disappointment, anger, emotional hurt, etc. Each of these *feelings* resulted from *your* negative thoughts. No matter what happens *outside your body*, only *what you think inside in your head* has the power to cause tension *inside your body*.

When you open one of those sticky doors into a room where you have stored tension, you are on the threshold of discovery! I encourage you to clean the room, by *forgiving* that someone, **even if it is you**, *letting go* of the grief, sadness, frustration, disappointment, anger, emotional hurt, etc., that has cluttered the room and closed the door. Know that those *feelings* are secondary emotions. Anger, pain, frustration, sadness, grief … all are negative feelings that are *secondary* emotions.

The *primary* negative emotion or feeling is *fear*.

Happiness, joy, peace, contentment are also secondary emotions or feelings.

The primary positive emotion or feeling is *love*.

People have two primary *thought* characteristics: positive and negative. And people have two primary *feeling* characteristics: love and fear.

Put your hand on the door. With positive thoughts (therefore filled with love), boldly enter each room, open the window and leave the door ajar, allowing the *clean air* to flow freely in from outside and into the rest of the house. Let go of the tension and its root cause: *fear*.

Know that only you were ultimately responsible for creating and storing the tension in your body.

You <u>*create*</u> <u>your own tension with your negative thoughts</u>.

No person, place, thing (or lack thereof) can create negative thoughts. Know that *only you* are responsible for *keeping the body filled with tension*.

Know that only you are responsible for releasing the tension that you created and stored in the body.

<u>You *release*</u> <u>your own tension with your positive thoughts.</u>

Know that *only you* are responsible for *keeping the body free of tension*. You have the power to keep each room clean.
You keep the body free of tension with your thoughts.
Only you have the power to create, store and release tension in your body.

You *can't* change or control other people or anything that has already happened outside your mind and body.

However, you can control your thoughts. Your thoughts control your feelings. Your feelings determine whether you feel love or fear. Your choice whether you ultimately feel love or fear determines whether *you* are creating or releasing tension.
Open the door and go in.
Believe that you can *clean* the room with your positive thoughts and the feelings of love that accompany your positive thoughts.

Practicing asanas while breathing full deep breaths will *train* your body to relax.

You can teach your body to relax when you have:

1. a desire to learn
2. your own words of encouragement and
3. a commitment to keep practicing

You can learn anything using those three magic ingredients.

Come back to your house. In the room where you discovered the tension, you will discover the person, place or thing that *you chose (or are still choosing) to perceive negatively* that is behind that tension, the fear.

With that same power to choose, choose to perceive that person, place or thing positively. With tension, the idea of "time" doesn't matter. It doesn't matter if the source of the tension is something that is in the past, present, or future. The body doesn't have a tension clock or calendar. Knowing this, it is then your job to create positive thoughts for that person, place or thing. That person, place or thing was put into your life to help you and has value. Ask yourself what can be learned and what can be valued. *You can* learn gentleness from an angry person. *You can* appreciate joy when living an unhappy place. *You can* see the value of what seems to be a useless thing. *You can* anticipate something good coming out of what seems to be an unpleasant-sounding upcoming event.

Read *Pollyanna*.

You can. I believe in you.

Mrs. Winings' belief in me was enough to instill my own belief in me. I understand now that I had the power to be my own Mrs. Winings all along; I just didn't know it at the time.

Mrs. Winings had a magic ability to awaken something in me. Would you like to know the secret behind her magic?

The Magic's Secret

I'm not a magician, so I can reveal the secret to her magic. Mrs. Winings awakened something in me that was already there.

She gave me **the key that unlocked something in my mind**.

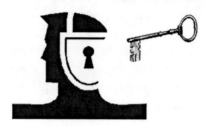

It doesn't matter what other people say to you.

What matters is what you say to you.

That is the **key**.

Your words, your feelings, your thoughts are what creates your experiences. The negative words and thoughts create the negative feelings, which create and attract the negative experiences. Negative feelings create tension. The positive words and thoughts create the positive feelings, which create and attract the positive experiences. Positive feelings promote the experience of joy. And joy releases tension.

Mrs. Winings said, "You really are a good writer. You are smart."

The *magic* occurred in me when the words changed in my own mind from her voice saying, "You really are a good writer. You are smart," to **MY OWN VOICE** saying, "I'm really a good writer. I am smart."

STOP! That is the magic's secret.

What matters is what you say to you.

Read the sentence above again. I wrote this book for this purpose: to tell other people about the magic's secret.

What matters is what you say to you.

In the end, it was *my own thoughts and feelings following* her words that made a difference.

Please, let me be your Mrs. Winings. Everyone has the power to be his or her own Mrs. Winings. That was her gift to me.

I understand now that Mrs. Winings is just a metaphor. Her voice is the voice of love and encouragement in the universe, the same voice that is inside **all** of us.

Can you hear her?

Choose Your Own Positive Thoughts

As you discover in your body the sources of tension, have *faith* that *you can* choose positive thoughts and feelings of love for this person, place or thing that you used to perceive with negative thoughts and those accompanying feelings of fear … and then patiently wait for those thoughts to come.

Make up positive thoughts about this person, place or thing, **even if you don't currently believe them to be true** and repeat them to yourself.

Make a space in your mind for those positive thoughts. "Listen" for them and believe that you will hear them in your own mind.

Believe you have the power to do this. **Everything in your life has a positive purpose.**

The negative thoughts you are repeating and holding on to *hurt*, don't they? Why are you hurting yourself? *You can make the hurting stop by changing your thoughts.*

You can change your perception of the whole world just by changing your thoughts. The world doesn't have to change at all. The definition of insanity is said to be thinking, believing or doing the same thing repeatedly and expecting a different outcome.

You're not crazy.

You are smart.

Now *you say it,* aloud or in your head, *in your voice.*

I am smart.

It feels good doesn't it? Say it again. I invite you now to say:

I am a positive person. I see the value in all the people, places, and things in my past, present and future worlds. Every person, place and thing has value and a purpose and I can always find something positive to think or say about everything. I think positively about the people, places and things in my past, present and future worlds. I think positively. I am a positive person.

Don't worry if you don't believe it at first. Keep saying it and eventually you will believe that it is true. The other things you're telling yourself aren't ever going to make you happy.

It becomes true in your mind when *you say it in your own voice* using I statements. However, just as you have willingly invested time in practicing saying the negative things, you must willingly invest time in saying the positive things.

Just as a steady stream of water *will* erode stone, a steady stream of positive thoughts has the power to dissolve tension and change your feelings. Eventually, that *channel* in the body becomes unblocked. Keep at it!

When you are practicing yoga, the asana, which used to find tension, eventually releases joy. Yoga's magic starts in the mind and then it is felt in the body.

The joy that flows through you is a gift, giving you the strength to clean your house. Joy provides you with those little daily victories over stored tension, giving you the courage to continue to discover, understand, and release tension.

Release tension, guided by the asanas, using your thoughts, your feelings and your breathing. Releasing tension releases joy.

Joy gives you the *juice* to promote positive feelings that charge you with positive thoughts and perceptions that help you *not* create *new tension* in the Now.

Three simple rules:

1. You can't have a negative thought if you're having a positive thought.
2. You can't release tension with a negative thought.
3. You can't create tension with a positive thought.

Chapter 8

The Chemistry of Yoga

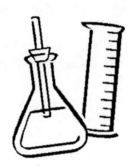

Repeated activation of the relaxation response can reverse sustained problems in the body and mend the internal wear and tear brought on by stress.
—HERBERT BENSON, MD

Fear is a question: What are you afraid of, and why? Just as the seed of health is in illness, because illness contains information, your fears are a treasure house of self-knowledge if you explore them.
—MARILYN FERGUSON

Just as stress releases chemicals in the body, joy releases its own powerful brand of chemicals; powerful chemicals that help dissolve pain and fill you with feelings of happiness.

These chemicals are the science behind yoga, for those who enjoy a connection with a scientific explanation.

These *joy* chemicals are also highly addictive and you will come to enjoy and crave them, which helps make it easier and easier to practice.

In the beginning, it requires effort and discipline to unroll your mat to practice. Eventually, the thought of *not* practicing yoga seems strange and unnatural.

Tension's Chemical Origin

So, how does tightness or tension get created and stored in the body in the first place?

Here is where the connection between the mind and the body and the wonderful chemistry linking them emerges.

How you think about the world is characterized as being either negative or positive. If through conditioning or other experiences, your thoughts tend toward negativity, those negative thoughts *generate* negative feelings that cause stress in the body. Negative thoughts *always* have at their root some fear or perceived threat to your security.

When you feel stressed due to some real or perceived threat to your security, you *feel* fear and **adrenaline** is released in the body. The release of adrenaline triggers the *flight or fight syndrome*, preparing the body for great physical exertion. A greater real or perceived threat results in a greater accompanying feeling of fear, since the amount of adrenaline secreted will be in direct proportion to the *intensity* of the fear-based feelings. So, a greater accompanying feeling of fear results in a greater amount of adrenaline being released into the muscles. The intensity of these fear-based feelings is *governed solely* by the intensity of the fear-based thoughts.

In situations and societies where running and/or fighting are inappropriate, the adrenaline, with no accompanying physical exertion to burn it off, creates poisonous by-products which are stored in the major muscle groups to which the adrenaline is distributed. The result is tension, tension proportionate to the amount of accumulated by-products.

Just as unexpended calories result in *stored fat*, unexpended adrenaline by-products result in *stored tension*.

Remember to label the underlying feeling behind the tension that occurs. The negative thoughts generate the feeling of *fear*. Your thoughts—and your thoughts alone—have the power to create feelings of fear. Real or perceived threats to your security, whether they are threats to your *physical* or *emotional* security, cause the release of adrenaline. Your body is simply obedient and does not know the difference between a real and *perceived* threat *or* the difference between your physical and your *emotional* security.

It is simple cause and effect:

a. you see something
b. your mind interprets that something as a threat, and
c. your body *feels* a discomfort called fear

Now, the *obedient* body takes over:

a. adrenaline is released to power the fight or flight, but
b. you don't run or fight because it's not appropriate in the situation, so no physical energy is expended, therefore,
c. adrenaline is released and with no accompanying physical exertion, the adrenaline by-products become a toxin in the body, which is stored in the major muscle areas, like the shoulders, neck, hips and legs

There's your tension.

Negative *memories* and *feelings* find "rooms" in the house or areas of the body to take up residence. All *like* memories and feelings store themselves in the same rooms. The body develops its own routine for processing your cycle of negative thoughts, negative feelings, proportionate adrenaline release, and storage location for the resulting tension. Eventually, these rooms become *cluttered* from these repeated negative thought, negative feeling, adrenaline release, and stored tension cycles. All the events and perception *memories and feelings* become part of the physical component matter of what makes your back, legs, neck, shoulder, etc. *feel* stiff or tense. Your "feelings" about you boss, dad, spouse, sense of isolation, etc., is in your stiff back, neck, hamstrings, or shoulders.

Living with this stiffness or tension and the accompanying pain, which, if prolonged enough, becomes like a pebble in your shoe and can be a constant nagging discomfort. Whole wings of your house become cluttered, and it affects your ability to love and be kind to your self and those with whom you come in contact.

Your pain, unless the people with whom you come in contact are enlightened beings who understand you and are actively removing tension from *their* bodies, *becomes their pain*.

Soon, there goes the neighborhood …

The Tension Cycle

Here is a summary of the Tension Cycle:

1. Negative thoughts create fear—as you perceive a threat to your physical, mental and/or emotional safety.
2. The fear response causes your body to release adrenaline.
3. Following the adrenaline release, you do not engage in any physical exertion.
4. The adrenaline by-products are stored in the muscles.
5. The stored by-products of adrenaline result in physical tension.
6. Physical tension creates negative thoughts and feelings ("I hurt, I'm stiff, I'm sore …").
7. Negative thoughts and feelings attract more negative thoughts and feelings.

A Bath of Compassion

While you are practicing, feel where you are tight in an asana. Is it your hips? Is it your shoulders, your arms, your waist, lower back, hamstrings, ankles, or neck? Welcome those discoveries of tightness with a mother's compassion! Imagine there is a part of you that has *witnessed* all your hurts, sufferings and fearful reactions (but *not* shared or felt them) since you were a child.

Imagine this *witness* has a mother's compassion and is bathing your body. Let your *witness* teach you and encourage you to take deep breaths, and imagine those deep breaths are clean water, cleansing and purifying those areas of tension.

Let the *witness* soothe you with comforting words of encouragement and love, love for your self and for the people who you discover in your thoughts when you feel tension.

Imagine that your arms, legs, neck and torso and all the places where you feel tension, simply need to be cleaned.

Acknowledge the tension is there and each time you breathe, *feel* the tension releasing; let it go. Dip the soiled area in the pure water of the breath. As you twist in an asana or sink into the depth of an asana, imagine that you are wringing out a cloth, and see the dirty water drip from your body and seep into the earth.

The Asana Cycle

Here is a summary of the Asana Cycle:

1. Deliberately creating the feeling of bliss (a relaxed face, imagining a "soft" body, smiling with a closed mouth, happy or "no" thoughts) while practicing asanas safely allows you to "discover" tension areas in the body.
2. The physical practice causes the body to release endorphins and other "feel good" chemicals into the blood stream.
3. Positive feelings during asanas, engaging bandhas to direct energy up the spine and deep breathing release tension during asanas.
4. Releasing tension creates a feeling of relief, promotes relaxation and that "joy" feeling.
5. The "joy" feeling attracts more joyful thoughts and feelings.
6. Positive thoughts and joyful feelings are associated consciously and unconsciously with practicing yoga.

Letting Go—It's Your Choice

Sometimes, in these moments of discovery and release, channels, previously blocked, become unblocked, and as a reward for your efforts, you feel joy.

Know that *your* thoughts of hurt, disappointment, pain, frustration, hatred, anxiety, etc., created the feelings of fear, caused the release of adrenaline, and resulted in the storage of tension. The tension you encounter through the asanas is all ultimately the result of *your negative thoughts*—thoughts that generated negative *feelings* or fear.

Tension is stored in your body through an uncomplicated biological process. Just like excess unburned calories become fat, excess negative emotions or feelings become tension.

It's so simple, but for some people, the pain they feel can remain a lifelong, elusive mystery. They believe that the cause is some person, place or thing in their past, present or future worlds. The sad thing is that they don't know *they are literally manufacturing the pain themselves.*

No one forces you to think.

It's said that our greatest power is our power to choose.

Why do we choose negative thoughts?

Negative thoughts generate negative *feelings.* Negative feelings generate tension—simple cause and effect.

Be Perfectly Selfish

Tension causes pain. Pain feels bad.

To be perfectly selfish, if you desire a life of ease and comfort, be selfish and choose positive thoughts, which generate positive *feelings*, which stimulate the release of **endorphins** and other chemicals that make the body feel good, and bring a gentle smile to the face. That's joy.

Joy causes happiness. Joy feels good.

If you find tension, and discover that behind it is a stored painful memory, maybe someone you need to forgive, grief, sadness,

41

hatred, frustration, anger or any other fear-based *things*, I invite you to let all these things go.

In order to change your feelings, you need to change your thoughts.

So you can feel happy.

Chpater 9

Be the Light Bulb / See the Light Bulb

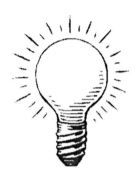

People are like stained-glass windows. They sparkle and shine when the sun is out, but when the darkness sets in their true beauty is revealed only if there is a light from within.
—ELIZABETH KUBLER-ROSS

There are two ways of spreading light: to be the candle or the mirror that reflects it.
—EDITH WHARTON, *Vesalius in Zante*

When you let your own light shine, you unconsciously give others permission to do the same.
—NELSON MANDELA

Anyone who ventures boldly into this internal world of discovery begins to release a powerful "current" of positive energy. This current of energy has the power to heal not only you, but it is *felt* and can *heal* those you with whom you come in contact.

Have you ever met a happy person? What do you *think* when you are around them? What do you *feel*?

How about an unhappy person? What do you *think* when you are around them? What do you *feel*?

Joy or love is like electricity, and you are like a light bulb. You give off *light* and feel *warmth* when you allow this electricity to *flow though* you.

Other people are attracted to your light. You become accustomed to the warmth.

By choosing thoughts of love, you are choosing to flip the switch that allows the current to flow. The bulb warms and glows brightly.

You begin to see that this electricity is everywhere, not just inside you, but also waiting inside everyone.

You see that everyone is a light bulb.

Some light bulbs need help before they can glow.

If you send enough love, through your positive thoughts, feelings and actions, your can encourage others to flip their switch and allow the electricity to flow through them.

This helps them see that everyone is a light bulb …

Yoga Can Be Practiced When You're Not Practicing Yoga

Eventually, the peace and tranquility you feel when you are done practicing yoga begins to last longer and longer, spilling over into the rest of each day.

You begin to see opportunities to practice yoga even when you are not physically practicing yoga, especially when you think.

Yoga means union. Connecting to that place of peace and tranquility inside you can happen when you are driving, preparing food, walking to the mailbox or simply sitting quietly and enjoying the sounds the day makes.

Chapter 10

Practice, Practice, Practice

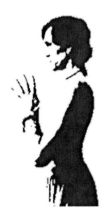

The ordinary acts we practice every day at home are of more importance to the soul than their simplicity might suggest.
—THOMAS MOORE

If it hurts, you are doing it wrong. Get your jam up and let your prana heal you. Who knows what will happen?

Make your experience of yoga as fun and pleasurable as possible, so that you look forward to it the next day.
—DAVID WILLIAMS

Yoga is the practice of quieting the mind.
—PATANJALI

Yoga is 99% practice and 1% knowledge.
—SRI KRISHNA PATTABHI JOIS

Wherever and whenever you practice, if you practice alone, make a special place to go each day where you won't be disturbed and practice.

Remember that as long as you live and breathe, each day you will encounter people and situations that present you with the opportunity to feel love or fear. Releasing old tension, breathing, relaxing, perspiring, and releasing joy is the best way to be prepared to offer your best to people and situations in the Now.

The quality, duration, and consistency of your practice directly relates to the amount of calmness, compassion, and feelings of love you are able to give to yourself and others.

If you **desire to learn** yoga or anything else, just add the other two magic ingredients: **encouragement** and **practice**.

I believe my yoga is only limited now by **practice**.

I have a desire to learn and have provided myself a steady diet of love and encouragement. Remember, the only love and encouragement *you* can be assured of receiving is that which you provide for yourself.

Above all, practice, practice, practice.

"Practice," as Pattabhi Jois says, "[and] all is coming."

Learning and Practicing Asanas

In the beginning, learning and practicing asanas is a *very conscious process*.

Asanas and series of asanas in the Ashtanga Yoga system are progressive, meaning each new asana "builds" on the postures, concepts, and movements developed in the previous asanas.

Learning and practicing asanas is like learning and practicing anything else.

Have you ever thought about *how* you learn?

Learning is a human behavior. Human behavior is a learned response. Learning is your perception, assimilation and application of external or internal information using your *thoughts, feelings* and *bodily responses to those thoughts and feelings.*

Your thoughts, feelings and bodily responses are all "wired" together or connected.

Using repetition or practice and *the magic of positive thinking*, actions performed very *consciously* or with a great deal of "thinking" in the beginning eventually become *unconscious* with very little accompanied thinking. After much repetition or practice, the body just "knows" how to do something with little conscious input from the brain. The body seems to "know" because it has performed these physical "actions" so many times.

Did you ever wonder how this works?

Imagine that in your brain, each individual step in any physical action or skill, like playing the piano, is broken down into a series of numbered steps, like in an instruction manual.

These numbered steps are punctuated in your brain by *dendrites* or little electrical terminations that connect the dots between a mental stimulus and physical action. When you are learning anything, the brain carefully sets out a trail of breadcrumbs or numbered steps so the electrical impulse can *remember* the path from the part of the brain that senses the mental stimulus to the part of the brain that triggers the associated physical actions or skills.

This is bioelectrical instruction manual is called the dendrite path.

Over time, through repeated trips down this path, the electrical impulse has to stop at fewer of the breadcrumbs along the path until eventually it goes directly from mental stimulus to the physical action. The dendrite path, like any well-traveled path, becomes worn and the electrical impulse no longer needs "breadcrumbs" to find its way. Behavior becomes automatic through repetition.

The behavior goes from being *very conscious* to being *unconscious*.

The only difference between someone who can beautifully play a Mozart piece on the piano and someone who looks at the piano and sheet music and says, "Huh?" is:

- the **desire to learn**,
- hundreds of hours of **practice**, and

- **words of encouragement**

Regarding encouragement, *the most important* words of encouragement are your own. If you do not have an official teacher then *you* are all you have.

What words do you use to describe your practice? Are they positive or negative?

Remember, negative words cause negative feelings, which result in tension in the body and will create more work for you.

Positive words release tension in the body and will make your practice easier. The key is to feel happy where you are.

Feeling happy and grateful about where you are currently will, by the Law of Attraction, bring you more things that make you feel happy and grateful.

THIS IS THE SECRET TO YOGA ... AND THE SECRET TO ATTRACTING MORE OF WHAT YOU WANT INTO YOUR LIFE!

Putting on Your Bliss Face

Let me take you further. Look deeply into your eyes in the mirror, smile with your lips closed and breathe deeply in and out. Now, slowly close your eyes while holding this look on your face and continue to breathe. When you practice, keep this look on your face! I've heard that it takes only 10 or so muscles to arrange your face into a smile and over 100 to arrange your face into a frown.

I've been in practice rooms and seen some grim looks on people's faces. I want to shout, THIS IS SUPPOSED TO FEEL GOOD!

If you already practice yoga, do you have a bliss face or do you look serious and in pain?

Yoga can help you feel good, if you will just allow that to happen. Make feeling good your intention each morning when you wake up, practice and go through your day.

Say, "I intend to feel good today!"

Put on your bliss face.

Arranging your face into a "look" of bliss fools your body into feeling happy. This will release "feel good" chemicals into the blood stream and acts as a rocket booster to helping you release tension and open the floodgates (the various channels in your body) to allow joy to flow unobstructed. Feel the old stored organic by-products of stress, emotional pain and other hurts melting away each time you practice.

When you wake up in the morning, put on your bliss face and begin to feel the effects it has on your body, your mind and your outlook on life. Notice how other people act when they encounter your bliss face.

Raising Your Frequency and Making Beautiful Crystals

In *Power vs. Force: The Hidden Determinants of Human Behavior*, author David Hawkins describes how different emotions have different frequencies. Hate and despair rank low and are among the destructive energies. Love and gratitude rank #1 and #2 as the highest frequency emotions.

Feelings attrached to thoughts are what create what you see in your life. Practice noticing your thoughts ... and feelings.

Thinking thoughts that create the feelings of love and gratitude while you do anything will attract to you more things that make you feel loving and grateful.

Thinking thoughts that create the feelings of anger, sadness, despair, grief, frustration, depression or any negative feelings will attract to you more things that create these emotions.

You are smart. If you don't believe me, the next time you're feeling bad, back up and review what you were just thinking. Behind any bad feeling you're experiencing is a trail of negative mental breadcrumbs.

See what I mean?

Remember though that positive feelings have a measurably higher frequency than negative feelings.

That means that positive feelings have a greater creative power or pull within the Universe to get you what you want.

Positive feelings have clout!

Feeling love and gratitude will fill you with the highest possible frequencies and energies and you will naturally attract more of the same.

Let's expand on this idea. In the book *The Hidden Messages in Water*, Dr. Masaru Emoto describes how he used high-speed photography to discover that crystals formed in frozen water change when specific, concentrated thoughts were focused toward them. Water from clean sources *and* water exposed to loving words showed beautiful, complex, and colorful snowflake patterns. On the other hand, polluted water, or water exposed to negative thoughts or words, formed broken patterns with drab colors. Think about the implications of this research creates.

What does this mean to you?

You are 70% water.

Think about Dr. Emoto's findings: Thinking thoughts that make you feel happy and grateful, that is those good thoughts that you direct toward your body's water in your current place in any pose not only attracts more things to make you feel happy and grateful into your practice, it attracts more into your life.

Feeling love and gratitude is an inside job.

Kathy and I have a beautiful glass two-gallon container of distilled water on our kitchen counter. We have made a sign that says "Love & Gratitude" and have taped it to the glass so the words face inward, directed toward the water. When we drink it, we know that we are drinking water that has the highest possible frequency and energy. I've put Love & Gratitude signs in our refrigerator, directed toward our food. When we eat, we know that we are eating food that has the highest possible frequency and energy. We love to have people over and share our home, our food, and our love and gratitude. When people eat food or drink water at our home, those two extra ingredients are included. They don't see them, they *feel* them.

Imagine then that your thoughts of love and gratitude, whether in a yoga pose or as you go through the motions of your day, are pieces of paper that you are directing toward the water that comprises 70% of the inside of your body. Washing clothes is yoga.

Driving your kids around is yoga. Eating is yoga. Sleeping is yoga. Listening to beautiful music is yoga. It's all yoga.

Let's say you need to bend your knees to bend forward and rest your palms on the floor. If you are unhappy that your knees are bent, UNHAPPY is a negative emotion, which is a by-product of a negative thought. The negative thought might be, "My knees should be straight," or you might hold in your mind the image of someone else more flexible doing the pose and comparing yourself to them and *feeling* less than.

Beware: Those negative thoughts and feelings directed toward your body's water in the pose are attracting more thoughts that are negative. Your yoga practice, which is intended to increase your joy, ends up being another part of your life you are not feeling good about.

Feel good while you practice.

The only way to feel good is to be thinking happy thoughts or just experiencing the thoughtless joy the comes when you have memorized the practice sequence and you are tuned in to the sound of your breath and feeling the good feelings that come when tension is released.

How do you know if you are thinking good thoughts? Simple: You will feel good. Good feelings follow good thoughts. Bad feelings and tension follow bad thoughts.

If you're doing yoga but thinking about all you have to do that day and feeling stressed out, you'll be doing what my beautiful wife Kathy calls PISSED OFF YOGA.

Consider these words:

"I have a hard time finding time to practice. I can't touch my toes. I'm not very flexible. *I'm stiff. I hurt.* I have no upper body strength. I'll never do a handstand, headstand, backbend, it hurts when I do this or *that*, etc."

Now, consider these:

"I look forward to practice every day. I'm closer to touching my toes than I was when I started. I feel myself getting more flexible.

My upper body is getting stronger. I enjoy trying to do a handstand, headstand, backbend, etc."

What kind of words do you use?

(Do you have back pain? I highly recommend the book *Healing Back Pain: The Mind-Body Connection*, by John Sarno.)

If you have a negative "teacher" in your head, *fire him or her immediately.* **Only use positive words** and train yourself to be a positive teacher.

Know that you can become your own positive teacher (or anything you want to be) with a desire to learn, your own encouraging words and practice.

Read uplifting books. Read affirmations. Everyday, with a mother's tenderness and care, prepare healthy, **positive word meals of love** and feed your mind a healthy diet of positive words. When you practice yoga and when you do anything else.

Do you know the sure way to check? How do you feel? Your feelings are the body's natural indicator of gauging how you are thinking.

Remember these simple rules:

- Positive thoughts make you feel good
- Negative thoughts make you feel bad
- You alone are the author of your thoughts

Water your own seeds …

Remember the importance of thoughts when learning! Take great care to use words of love and encouragement during your practice and to describe your practice.

Becoming Consistent

Ashtanga tradition encourages a daily practice, but invites its practitioners to take off Saturdays and each month's new and full moon days.

Consider adopting these Saturday and moon days off in to your practice. Consider these "days off" to be just as important as "days on" and enjoy them as a part of, not separate from, your practice.

On the practice days, try and practice, even if your practice that day is comprised of only a few Sun Salutations and Shavasana. Build up over time.

Practicing at the same time every day is a good way to habituate yourself to the joy of your practice. Consider eventually practicing in the morning.

Yes, the morning.

When you read, "The morning," what did you think? Were your thoughts positive or negative? I confess that when I considered practicing in the morning, my mind used to fire off a series of negative, self-defeating thoughts that produced tension in my body.

Can you imagine?

The thought of practicing in the morning, when the body is at its "stiffest" seems impossible. However, when I practiced during my lunch hour or tried to squeeze it in here and there, other responsibilities would often materialize that required my time and I would end up "missing" those opportunities to practice.

I began to observe the change in me when I practiced "regularly" and made up my mind to make practice a regular part of each day. The only time of day that seemed immune to interruption was the early morning.

But, my love for yoga had grown so I agreed with myself that I would adjust to the morning. Not knowing what I was doing, I changed my thoughts, which changed my feelings, which released (or at least didn't create more) tension. I realized I had created morning phobia (fear) with my negative thoughts. Actually, changing to a morning yoga practitioner turned out to be the best thing that could have ever happened to me! After a few years, and through the miracle of health that yoga unleashes, I found that I required less and less sleep, and began to *enjoy* waking up while it was still dark to prepare for practice.

I discovered there is something magical about the morning. And the consistency with which I practiced began to grow.

But I certainly didn't start that way.

Work slowly and with great patience. You have your whole life ahead of you to practice. If you can't practice on a particular day, please don't panic or feel bad.

When you miss practice, with a mother's compassion, encourage yourself to practice at the next opportunity. Forgive yourself if you are feeling guilty or better, the moment you begin to recognize negative, self-defeating thoughts. Love yourself, even on days you don't/can't practice. Remember that today's guilt is tomorrow's tension. Resolve not to create more "work" for your *next* practice.

Keep picturing yourself practicing regularly. Imagine that this picture is a beautiful lily in bloom in a stream at your feet. Stare at it. Appreciate it. Other thoughts, thoughts of fear, might pass by in the water, like sticks and old leaves.

Stare at the lily until you hardly notice the sticks and leaves. Picture the sticks and leaves disappearing and eventually, they stop floating by.

Eventually, all you'll see is the lily and you will be practicing in the morning.

If, like me, the morning is your only guaranteed time to consistently practice, consider it. Think about the Tension Cycle and the power your own thoughts have to create tension or release tension. Tell yourself you are a morning person and that you love starting each day with your yoga practice. Imagine you are writing the dialog for an actor that practices yoga in the morning with a wonderful regularity. In the "script," the actor is telling a friend about overcoming the "fear" of practicing in the morning:

"I love to wake up early each day to practice yoga. I used to think this was impossible, because I was stiff and unmotivated in the morning. I told others and myself that I 'wasn't a morning person'. Then I realized that my own thoughts and words had 'programmed' an exaggerated physical manifestation of stiffness and the feeling of 'not being a morning person' into me.

The hardest part in the beginning was waking up. After a while, by carefully monitoring my thoughts, I found I didn't even need an alarm clock any more!

Now, I look forward to my practice each morning. I wake up happy and get up immediately. I don't count the hours I've slept or 'program' myself to feel sleepy later in the day. I tell myself I will feel good when I wake up and that feeling will last all day. Upon rising, my muscles begin to warm as I consciously focus on relaxing and deep breathing. I feel my body begin to loosen and look forward to practice.

And because I make the time to practice each morning, I rarely miss practice.

I now consider myself a morning person.

Read the above dialog again. Read it aloud. *If you are willing to learn, it can be you saying it.* If I can do it, anyone can. Remember, I "scripted" the above for myself first and then eventually, it went from a script to reality. I changed my behavior by changing my thoughts. Changing my thoughts changed my feelings.

Make a space in your thoughts for thoughts of you being a morning person and they will come.

I wrote the above before practice one morning at what some would label a "God-awful hour."

I remember thinking it was a "magical" time of day. The house was quiet except for the musical clicking of the keys on the computer as I typed. I was listening to one of the CDs I play when I practice yoga. As I typed, I was imagining someone reading my words, changing their thoughts, and discovering the joy of the mornings.

I remember feeling very happy.

What I Practice

This is a personal choice.

Some days, my body might just need a little practice. I can always find time to do Shavasana (lying on my back with my feet shoulder-width apart, arms at my sides, palms turned up) for five minutes. David Williams told me that, as a minimum practice, he does the following:

- 3 Sun Salutation A's
- 3 Sun Salutation B's
- the last three Finishing Postures
- Corpse Posture

I've never practiced and regretted it.

Let your body tell you. Listen. There's no race. There's no point system awarded.

Be kind to your body and that kindness will return to you.

Let me tell you about my experience as an example of my own experimentation. Your mileage may vary, as the saying goes.

In the beginning, as I mentioned, I followed the Bryan Kest tapes. That seemed ok at the time.

Later, I followed Richard Freeman's tapes, but it took a long time and I found it hard to go from a 45-minute Bryan Kest tape to a 2-hour Richard Freeman tape, plus, anyone who's seen Richard Freeman's Primary Series tape might be very intimidated.

I was. (It wasn't you, Richard, it was my thoughts when watching you. I now understand this perfectly.)

Don't be intimidated. You aren't competing with Richard. You are seeing the fruit of his practice.

On his website, Richard mentions that an option, for the time constrained, is to break the practice down each week, for example, as follows:

DAY 1: Sun Salutations A & B, Standing Postures, Finishing Postures, Shavasana
DAY 2: : Sun Salutations A & B, Seated Postures, Finishing Postures, Shavasana
Day 3: Repeat Day 1
Day 4: Repeat Day 2
Day 5: Repeat Day 1
Day 6: Repeat Day 2
Saturday: Off

Add days off on Saturdays and on the full and new moon days, but keep to the alternate Standing and Seated Postures method. That way, each week, you are exposing your body to a "complete" Primary Series several times.

Eventually, you may find the strength to go all the way through the Primary Series each day. Or maybe, one day a week when you have more time and energy, like Sunday, you can attempt the whole Primary Series. Some days, you might only do Shavasana. Say, "I practice yoga every day."

Remember, there's no race or point system.

I used the above to work towards doing the Primary Series each day. I took my time, didn't set a deadline, and when my body was ready, I was able to do what I used to think was impossible. I said, "I practice the full Primary Series every day," even before it was true.

It happened so slowly. The flexibility, strength, endurance, and balance all built themselves in tiny increments.

I made a space in my mind for thoughts of me doing the whole Primary Series.

Wherever you are in your yoga journey, write the script for where you will go, and watch all those marvelous changes begin to happen.

And remember to make a space in your mind for the changes.

Give yourself permission to picture yourself doing someday what you might think impossible now. Program yourself with positive words and thought pictures. Watch your positive words and thought pictures become reality.

Let them become reality slowly and leave the calendar and stop watch behind. Your words and thought pictures have their own timing. The wonderful changes that come along with them will be appreciated and valued by you if they happen slowly and feel like something you earned yourself.

There's no race, rush or points system in yoga. Just you and your wonderful body.

Nearly this entire book was written before each morning's practice. I believe it, because it happened to me, but there is still a part of me thinking, "Wow, I actually did it!" After Christine's invitation to narrate my practice was converted in my mind into the idea of compiling all those asana descriptions into a "book," I wondered when I would find the time to write. When I looked at my scheduled, I *believed* that the morning *before* I practiced yoga would be the best time. Luckily, I just acted on that belief and did not check with others, who would have surely told me that waking up in the middle of the night, writing for many hours, practicing yoga, and then going to work all day would result in sickness or possibly death. I did not get sick. I didn't die. I find that I have to be very careful about sharing ambitious goals. You will not have to travel far to find someone to "talk" you out of a goal. Keep your goals quiet and always be your own coach and mentor. Let the only voice of encouragement you ever need to hear be your own. You are always available to you. I wrote most of the first draft of this book in the span of about one month. I *believed* that writing this book would make me happy (since the book was finally coming out, as Jeff's cartoon suggested). I also *believed* that writing would give me more mental and physical energy, just like when you are a little happy kid playing for hours tirelessly at something that brings you joy. Though I have experienced this "believe and see" phenomenon repeatedly in my life, each time it happens, I am still amazed.

If you think, "Well this whole positive thinking and 'believe and see' business works for Danny only *because he believes it*," you are right. *Believe it can work for you* and you will be right again.

Chapter 11

True Confession: I Pour Warm Saltwater in My Nose

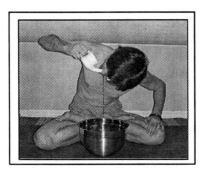

Though this be madness, yet there is method in it.
—WILLIAM SHAKESPEARE

As far as yoga goes, 99% of the breathing involves air entering and leaving the body through the nostrils. Your nostrils and immediate interior of the nose are equipped with a simple filtration system to trap airborne dirt and particles.

Many diseases and sicknesses start with impurities that enter the nostrils. Daily neti pot cleansing helps keep the nose clean and improves overall health. Cleansing the nose in this manner allows the breath to move more easily in and out of the body.

A neti pot looks like a small teapot with an elongated spout. Neti pots are avaible online, at some pharmacies or at health food stores and are relatively inexpensive.

A neti pot's primary feature is the diameter of the end of the spout, designed to be small enough to insert into the nostrils.

You will be pouring a mild saline solution into one nostril and, because of the angle at which the head is held, the water will drain out the other nostril. With the body bent at the waist over a sink, with your elbow on the counter, gravity does not permit the water to run down the back of the throat into the lungs—which is what I was afraid of when I first heard about this. You are merely pouring warm water (with a hint of salt) into one nostril and out the other in order to flush out the trapped dirt and particles.

Note: Have faith! The first time you try this, it doesn't seem like it will work, but then you see the water pouring out the other nostril and your belief system kicks in.

There is a central passage above each nostril. Think of an inverted letter Y. A short distance into your nose, there is a place where the mild saline solution can find a way into the other nostril and out of the body.

How to Use a Neti Pot

1. Put 1/8th of a teaspoon of uniodized salt into the neti pot.
2. Fill the neti pot with lukewarm water.
3. Lean over the sink and tip your head to the side as if to look up at the sky up over your right shoulder, but stare at your nose.
4. Hold the pot in your right hand and insert the spout in your right nostril.
5. Open your mouth and breathe in and out with the mouth throughout.
6. Lift your right elbow up to point at the ceiling slowly and start pouring.
7. Initially, the water meets resistance, but then it finds the path of least resistance (that central passage connecting the two openings) and it starts to flow out the left nostril.
8. Continue pouring until the water has all drained and the neti pot is empty. Relax and watch the water coming out.
9. Set the neti pot down. Keeping your mouth open, press your right nostril closed from the outside of the nose with your right index finger and gently "blow" air out the left nostril. The excess water and "dirt" should expel into the sink.

10. Repeat on the other side, pressing the outside of the left nostril with the left index finger, gently "blowing" air out the right nostril. The excess water and "dirt" should expel into the sink.

11. Refill the neti pot with warm water and 1/8th of a teaspoon of salt and repeat all the above steps. This time, look up toward the sky over your left shoulder, inserting the neti pot's spout in the left nostril and pour the solution so it drains out the right nostril, then "blow" your nose as described in steps 9 and 10 above.

Note: When you "blow" your nose after cleansing, keep your mouth open and blow gently so as not to put undo pressure on the ears.

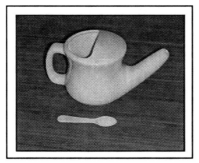

All you need is a neti pot, uniodized salt and a little spirit of adventure!

Chapter 12

Bandhas: The Master Keys to Yoga

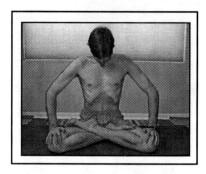

If I have ever made any valuable discoveries, it has been owing more to patient attention, than to any other talent.
—ISAAC NEWTON

Every asana has bandhas hidden within it. Bandhas ("locks") are one of yoga's paradoxes.

For the first two years of my practice, I knew about the bandhas, but ignored them.

I promise you, they are well worth focusing on!

The bandhas are probably the most important bodily concept in yoga practice next to breathing.

In the beginning, there is an understandable tendency in yoga to focus on the physical appearance of the postures. At first, it is a simple matter of trying to remember the general configuration of the body to "form" the asana.

Once the body is comfortable "forming" the basic asana, "finding" the bandhas, maintaining the even "quality" of the breath and remaining calm *within* the asana becomes the next layer of awareness.

Lastly, when the asanas, bandhas, and breath are natural, the mind is free to explore what is behind "found" tension and can aid in releasing joy through the construction of positive thoughts and eventually, to float freely in the joyful bliss of just being and doing, without any need to think (or overthink) at all.

For a while, I was stuck in the asana formation stage. The breath, bandhas and metaphysical exploration of my mind and body were not even in the equation in the beginning.

Now, I have found that the bandhas and the breath are actually more important and have found more enjoyment in my practice when I focus my intention less on the postures and more on the bandhas and breath. More enjoyment means more *in-joy-ment*, which keeps me unrolling my mat each day.

Paradoxically, yogic texts refer to bandhas as "locks," but I think they are more like little "keys" that open up great treasures in each practice.

How I Grew an Inch Taller

My son Andy came home from high school one day and told me that they had measured his height in gym class.

"How tall are you?" I asked.

"Six three," he said.

"But you're shorter than I am and I'm six three," I told him.

"Well, I'm six three. You must be at least six four," he told me.

Impossible! A doctor had measured me at 6' 3" several years ago following the car accident that had injured my back.

My driver's license says 6' 3".

How could I have grown an inch?

Maybe it was the work of the Uddiyana and Mula Bandhas.

I had started "holding" my spine straighter by making the longest possible line between the bottom of my sternum and the top of my pubic bone, with my upper chest pushed out and my shoulders dropped back. I began to hold myself as if I was "presenting" or holding my heart up and out for the world to see, which, now that I consider it, I was in more ways than I understood at the time.

The more I practiced the bandhas the less I had to "think" about "holding" myself in this posture.

It became more comfortable for me to "hold" myself this way and eventually, like all yoga practice, I started to practice what I practiced even after practice was over each day. It started to become automatic behavior.

A psychologist would say I had been unconsciously "shortening" the distance between the bottom of my sternum and the top of my pubic bottom because I was a self-conscious, fearful person. He would say unconsciously, I was drawing my shoulders inward and my ribs down to cover my vital organs and protect my heart. He might also say because I was self-conscious about feeling too tall, I had internalized other people's teasing about my height and I was unconsciously trying to appear smaller by slumping. He might also say that I was self-conscious about being too skinny and that I had internalized other people's teasing about my weight and I was unconsciously trying to appear "fatter" by slumping to push the muscles and skin on my abdomen outward.

A doctor would say I "grew" an inch taller because I was sitting and standing up straighter. He would say I had developed better posture.

A yoga teacher would say I had learned the Uddiyana and Mula Bandhas.

Mrs. Winings would say I was offering the world my heart.

Bandhas 101

Rather than describe each of the major bandhas, I will instead describe Maha Bandha (the Great Lock) which is the application of all three primary bandhas simultaneously.

It was easier for me to learn the three primary Bandhas through the application of Maha Bandha, as I found the spinal alignment from Maha Bandha held the "key" to understanding the physical subtleties of the Mula, Uddiyana and Jalandhara Bandhas:

1. In a standing position, draw yourself up to your fullest height, imagine the opposing forces as the feet simultaneously ground and sink into the earth like the roots of a tree and the crown of the head lifts higher and higher into the sky.
2. Imagine an "electrical" connection to the earth, from the soles of the feet that travels up through the crown of the head.
3. Bring your hands to the hips.
4. Keeping your back straight, bend your knees and spread your feet out and apart about 18-24 inches.
5. Turn the outer edges of the feet parallel by turning the toes in slightly.
6. Lift and curl back the toes to grip the earth gently.
7. With your hands on your hips, index fingers level with the top of your pubic bone and your thumbs on the rear of your hips, begin inhaling while you:
    - pull up the bottom of the spine, focusing internally at the base of the perineum (or cervix), imagine you are pulling the spine from the top of your head, pulling and imagining a space growing between every vertebra from the tip of the tail bone up into the top-most vertebra in the neck until at last, when the spine can be stretched no longer, the whole spine moves "up" and a tiny depression forms at the perineum (in males) and cervix (in females) as the tip of the spine is drawn away from the earth (Mula Bandha)
    - lift the sternum as high as you can and imagine making the maximum length between the bottom of the sternum and the top of the pubic bone—with this lengthening of the abdominal wall lift and spread the bottom of the rib cage, flaring the bottom-most ribs outward, and imagine feeling the skin on the shoulders and upper back sliding downward an inch over the muscles and bones (Uddiyana Bandha)
    - pull up through the top of the sternum, feeling the hollow at the base of the neck reach up toward the chin and

when it moves incline the head forward with no strain in the back of the neck—raising the sternum up to touch the chin while simultaneously pushing up and out through the top of the crown of your head (Jalandhara Bandha)

- exhale slowly with the tongue relaxed and the roof of the mouth soft and teeth apart until all the air leaves the body, but do not move your stomach and minimize the amount your ribs collapse as the lungs empty
- momentarily hold this engagement of all three Bandhas to create Maha Bandha
- go the extra mile and touch your tongue *gently* to the soft palette on the roof of your mouth (Jivha Bandha) right behind your top front teeth

8. Your dristi (gaze) is on the nose.
9. Your skin on your stomach stretches tight between the bottom of your ribs and the pubic bone.
10. Lift high with your chest, and imagine your heart itself is lifting and opening like a rose.
11. The shoulders blades keep dropping back and down in response to the chest's lifting action.

Note: During my entire practice, I hold the Mula and Uddiyana Bandhas until the end when I relax in Shavasana. I hold and release Jalandhara Bandha as directed. In each asana, there is at least one moment when I engage Maha Bandha*.

* Christine and I exchanged some emails about the idea of Maha Bandha in each asana. I was certain that there was a momentary engagement of Maha Bandha in each asana. No one told me this, I just noticed myself doing it. She disagreed and didn't want me to print something "wrong." She ended up writing to Sharath, Pattabhi Jois's grandson who responded, "Tell him he's right." To me it was not an item to debate the rightness or wrongness of, it was some-thing that occurred naturally in my practice that I observed. That momentary engagement of all three bandhas caused me to focus on taking my spine to it's maximum length. That's all. And since this

is a book about my practice, it's included, free of charge. Your mileage may vary.

Mula Bandha

Of all three bandhas, Mula Bandha was the trickiest for me to learn.

In all the reading I did, I learned that Mula Bandha is a slight contraction, in males, of the perineal body. I discovered that there's three muscle areas "down there" that you can contract:

1. The urogenital muscles, or the muscle you contract to interrupt the flow of urine.
2. The anal sphincter, or the muscle you contract to prevent gas escaping your body.
3. The muscle in between, which is located on the perineal body, which on males is between the anus and the genitals. On females, this area is located by contracting the cervix.

A good way to practice this is by doing what I call the 123 exercise. To do the 123 exercise, sit comfortably in a chair or cross-legged on the floor, so that you can straighten your spine. To straighten your spine, tuck you chin slightly and lift as high as you can through the crown of the head, press your belly in and flare your ribs out. You've just engaged the Jalandhara (neck) and Uddiyana (stomach) Bandhas.

1. Holding this position, inhale deeply, and exhale fully. When your breath is all the way out, contract and release your urogenital muscle. Call that contraction # 1.
2. Keep holding your Uddiyana and Jalandhara Bandhas. Inhale deeply, and exhale fully and retain the exhale. With your breath all the way out, contract and release your anal sphincter. Call that contraction # 3.
3. Keep holding Uddiyana and Jalandhara Bandhas. Inhale deeply, and exhale fully and retain the exhale. With your

67

breath all the way out, contract and release the urogenital muscle. Then contract and release the anal sphincter; then imagine "lifting" the muscle in between. When you "feel" that in-between muscle, make sure you don't feel a twitch or contraction in either the urogenital muscle or anal sphincter. Call that "in-between" muscle # 2.

4. Keep trying this same sequence, isolating and contracting #1, #2 and #3 until you can isolate #2 (Mula Bandha) without feeling a twitch in #1 or #3. You don't have to do it "hard" or create a painful feeling, it should be more of an awareness of that area of the body. While you're practicing yoga, you keep your awareness or attention there.

Rome was not built in a day. Since you've probably suppressed gas (#3) and interrupted the flow of urine (#1) many times during your life, those two muscle contractions will be stronger and easier to do. Learning to contract the "in-between" muscle (perineum for men and cervix for women) is new and will require a little work, but I promise it is worth it.

Focusing your attention on this muscle area or engaging Mula Bandha, and having your awareness in this area of the body activates tons of energy in the physical, mental and spiritual bodies. Energy naturally moves down the spine, but by engaging or holding Mula Bandha and Uddiyana Bandha, the energy is squeezed up into the solar plexus and heart and can aid in calming the mind during practice or at any time.

As you practice asanas, you will be discovering areas of tightness or tension in your body. These areas of tension were created from by-products of fear, so as you explore them, in order to safely move through and dissolve them, you need to move the energy up your spine, which will help dissolve those blockages (See Chapter 5, Your Body is a House and Chapter 6, The Chemistry of Yoga). Engaging Mula and Uddiyana Bandhas, putting on your Bliss Face and breathing deeply will help you relax and dissolve that organic tension.

The Master Keys

In yoga, much of the Sanskrit terminology, when translated, seems to describe something about the asana, either the part of the body being stretched or being "held."

Bandhas are called locks, as in *lock* this into place when performing asanas.

When I used to try and lock or hold Uddiyana Bandha during an asana, I shortened the distance between the bottom of my sternum and the top of my pubic bone and contracted my abdominal muscles.

For Mula Bandha, I read that Mula Bandha was applied by using the same muscles as were used to control/interrupt the flow of urine, so I made a gross muscular contraction of "those" internal muscles that did this. Later, I learned that it's also an anal contraction, so that had me puckering up to boot.

For Jalandhara Bandha, with my slumped posture, my shoulders rounding inward and clinching my urine and anal muscles, as the bottom of my sternum moved downward toward the top of the pubic bone, I would strain my chin forward until I could touch the top of my sternum.

All three bandhas were extremely uncomfortable.

The discomfort caused tension. When I thought about bandhas, read about bandhas and especially performed bandhas, I created negative thoughts.

I have a confession: I hated bandhas! I hated every one of them. I hated Mula first, Uddiyana second and Jalandhara third. But I hated Maha Bandha *most*, because it meant doing all three at once, which put me in the greatest amount of discomfort.

It was like getting my driver's license renewed, getting a tooth drilled and doing my taxes *all at the same time*.

I kept reading how important bandhas are … and my mind fired off a series of negative thoughts each and every time I read that.

So I kept practicing. I believed that bandhas must be important, because every single practitioner seemed to be *over emphasizing* their importance.

It was impossible to omit them.

I suddenly had a real **desire to learn** the bandhas.

This desire to learn made a space in my mind to learn bandhas. That meant that all I was missing was some of the steps. I knew, like anything else, once I had the steps, it was just a matter of practice, repetition and wearing down dendrites.

I read one of the rare articles by David Williams and it was all about the bandhas and the breath.

That simple two-page article on Yoga Journal's website was probably one of the most influential yogic things I have read.

Search Yoga Journal's website for David Williams and you will find it. Read it.

He mentioned that he practiced nauli everyday. I *believed* the great David Williams, the man who brought Ashtanga Yoga to me, indirectly.

It wasn't until I discovered nauli that I got it.

The link to the site I sent to Christine showed a picture of a man demonstrating nauli.

The picture showed a man with his rib cage pushed all the way out and a long line between the bottom of his sternum and the top of his pubic bone.

The site described the position of the torso as Uddiyana Bandha and I got it.

Once I got Uddiyana Bandha, my thoughts changed from negative to positive about Uddiyana Bandha. Then, my thoughts about the other Bandhas changed from negative to positive.

- My own positive words were the **encouragement** I needed.
- I became filled with a **desire to learn** the Bandhas and their application.
- I began to **practice** nauli (and the Bandhas) in earnest.

Eventually, the bandha dendrite path began to wear down. My breathing grew stronger. My asanas became more comfortable, as Patanjali said they should be.

The bandhas are not *locks*. The Bandhas are *keys*.

The master keys.

Chapter 13

Your Breath is the Conductor ... Your Body, the Orchestra

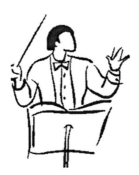

Smile, breathe and go slowly.
—THICH NHAT HANH

Breathing is an *unconscious* or autonomous bodily function, meaning we don't have to think about it for it to work. But unlike many other unconscious or autonomous bodily functions, breathing can be controlled *consciously*.

In yoga, a specific type of breathing is used called Ujjayi (victorious) breathing.

With each inhalation and exhalation cycle, a great volume of air is drawn deeply into the body and expelled. The stomach, because of the great distance between the bottom of the sternum and the pubic bone in each of the asanas, is flattened. Not sucked in using a muscular contraction and a shortening of the distance between the bottom of the sternum and the top of the pubic bone, but stretched and flattened through the deliberately exaggerated elongation of the spine.

With the torso held this way, the ribcage, therefore, moves in and out to accommodate the air, not the stomach.

The "sound" the air makes as it moves over the glottis is a deep, sibilant rasp.

The sound is made regular, musically speaking, and sounds the same whether the air is on its way in or out.

The length of time it takes to draw the air in or let it out is about five seconds from beginning of inhalation to end and from beginning of exhalation to end.

Inhale: 1, 2, 3, 4, 5
Exhale: 1, 2, 3, 4, 5

Conscious deep breaths release tension, and each time tension is released you feel a small sense of victory: victorious breathing.

Ujjayi Breathing is accomplished with a focus on the physical posture, attentiveness to the Bandhas, and a musician's ear for the even sound and duration of each cycle of your breath. Try it:

1. Engage Maha Bandha.
2. With the lips closed and smiling slightly, the tongue lies relaxed in the mouth, in its own tiny Shavasana.
3. The tip of the tongue moves forward to relax the tongue and lightly touches the area of the mouth right behind the tips of the front teeth.
4. The lips are closed but not pressed together and the teeth are not touching.
5. The palette is hollow, soft, and relaxed away from the tongue.
6. Without releasing the Maha Bandha (which means the stomach won't move), take a long slow deep breath in and try making an audible sound as the air passes over the glottis. The air's sound is a hollow, low-pitched rasp.
7. Out of your peripheral vision, see the ribs expand outward to accommodate the air.

8. Imagine that the breath travels into the nostrils, going all the way down to the tailbone.
9. Let out a long slow deep exhale and with a musician's ear make the exhalation *sound* the same as the inhalation.
10. Out of your peripheral vision, see the ribs collapse slightly inward as the air is released.
11. As you exhale, imagine the breath journeys back up the spine and out the body—your stomach stays stretched and still throughout.
12. The breath is strong and steady; the sound a gentle wind, the duration of each long, slow inhale is the same duration of each long, slow exhale.

Pay special attention to the quality of each inhale and exhale and try to fill and empty the lungs each time—concentrating on both the depth and regularity of sound.

When you incorporate the breathing in with the asanas, try and make each inhale and exhale last the duration of the movement within each asana or transitional movement between each asana.

Think of the breath as the conductor and the body as the orchestra. Move the body in time with the breath and not the other way around.

Try and make each movement, from beginning to end, last five slow counts, and hear the delicious rasping hiss of either the inhale or exhale that conducts the symphony of the body.

Chapter 14

Learning the Freaky Stomach Exercise

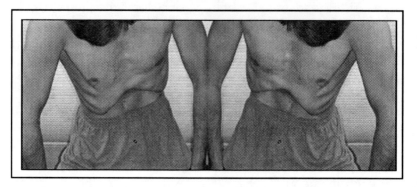

Keeping your body healthy is an expression of gratitude to the whole cosmos—the trees, the clouds, everything.
—THICH NHAT HANH

David Williams told me if he could only do one yogic thing, it would be nauli. He feels, health-wise, it is that important. He said he incorporates it into every day, like brushing his teeth.

Practicing nauli requires patience, but you will get the health benefits along the way, even if you never get your stomach to do those freaky flip-flops.

The time I visited David in Maui, he showed me his nauli. I watched in fascination as his stomach undulated back and forth, moving in a wave from one side of his abdominal cavity to the other in some ancient yogic hula.

Nauli is wonderful cleansing tool and helps develop the harmonious application of the Mula, Uddiyana, and Jalandhara Bandhas, or Maha Bandha (engaging all three bandhas in concert). Nauli also serves to warm the body, sending blood and oxygen into the muscles, making it a perfect beginning prior to any practice with it's unique focus on breath control, postural alignment, and the joy that comes when relaxing and discovering one of yoga's gifts.

With the feet 18-24 inches apart, bend the knees slightly.

1. Press the palms evenly into the tops of the thighs up near the head of the thighbone, where the thigh meets pelvis.
2. Place yours fingers together and arrange them so they are on the insides of your thighs and your thumbs are on the outside, with the heels of your hands facing your knees, while your thumbs and fingers "point" back toward your hips. Alternatively, you may place your palms down lower on the tops of the thighs, with the fingers and thumbs pointing toward the knees, thumbs on the inside of the thighs.
3. With your knees remaining bent, drop your chin in Jalandhara (lift your neck to its maximum length then drop the chin into the notch above the sternum; don't press down and compress your wind pipe, gradually lift and expand the chest and sternum to touch the chin ... without any constriction or tightness in the throat.)
4. Relax you mouth and allow the lips to touch each other with the lightest pressure, the teeth not touching.
5. Allow the tongue to rest softly in its own tiny Shavasana, as your palette relaxes into a quiet roof high above the tongue.
6. Lift through the perineum, engaging Mula Bandha.
7. Try and imagine creating the longest linear distance between the bottom of the sternum and the top of the pubic bone, pushing down evenly with your palms and out and up with your chest. Your rib cage should feel fully expanded.
8. Exhale completely through the mouth until all the air is out of your lungs.

Bottomline? The key to Bandhas & the nauli exercise in my mind is the Uddiyana Bandha. I believe my words can help anyone successfully "lock" in to Uddiyana Bandha. Let me tell you the "trick" in a brief explanation:

- Blow all the air out of your body … I mean every last bit
- Puff out your rib cage as far as you can (with ALL the air still out of your body)
- Move your shoulders down and back as far as you can

You should feel like your abdomen is "glued" to your back when you "get" this, since this "airless" lung state allows you to create a "vacuum" in the chest cavity that pull the stomach wall backwards.

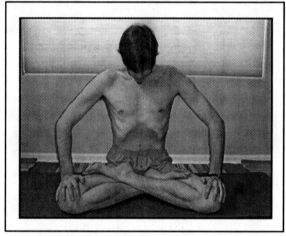

Blow __all__ the air out of your body then puff your ribcage out

Practice Udiyana Bandha until you can comfortably get into and "hold" your body in an Uddiyana Bandha, and then you are able to breathe and move your body in your yoga practice in a totally relaxed, fluid manner—with a mind and body in a state that you would describe as happy. Your ribs will still stay puffed out, your shoulders down and back and your chest lifting. In this gentle squeezing of the abdomen mode, it is much simpler, in my mind, to then bring my awareness to the Mula Bandha. This is the attitude of body and the state of mind with which the yogi seeks "no thoughts," whether it's in a meditative seated posture or while moving in and out of yoga poses with the bandhas gently "squeezing" against the spine held at it's maximum straightened length. The body and mind are relaxed, with a state of mind and body often described as happy, but *without the movement of thoughts through the mind*. The gentle, relaxed physical activation of the bandhas causes the associated muscle groups to stimulate the nerve plexuses, which cause the body to move electrical energy deliberately "up" the spine, which "feels" really good.

Bliss.

It's the reason you do yoga. To feel bliss. It's what you are on the Planet to experience. Try it and see what I mean.

Return to bliss each time you "practice" and work up to being able to put your self in this state when you wake up in the morning … then try and hold it all day long. If you practice anything enough, you can get it right? Come on, this is the one thing you can practice all day long. Bliss. Think about it. If people ask you, "Hey, why are you always smiling?"

Tell them to read my book.

FIRST PHASE:

This may be enough in the beginning. With all the air still exhaled, without straining the neck, try "lift" the abdominal muscle mass up and to the center and then relax it and let it "sag" down, so it looks like you are "bouncing" the mass up and down like a basketball using small muscular contractions. Try working up to 50 "bounces." Inhale, exhale and repeat up to five times.

SECOND PHASE:

When you have gotten stronger, after you exhale all the air out, try alternately pressing down the left palm firmly into your thigh, then the right palm, and watch as the abdominal mass "shifts" from side to side. "Shift" from left to right and back, back and forth … one … back and forth two … up to 50 times and repeat this up to five times. Inhale and exhale all the air out in between and always perform nauli exercises with the body in an airless state. If you want, you can try doing this seated in a chair. Try this in private without a shirt on so you can watch what's happening down there.

THIRD PHASE:

When "bouncing" and "shifting" have become comfortable, concentrate on moving the abdominal mass in a "churning" motion, first clockwise, then counter clockwise, in up to 50 tiny circles in each direction, five times each side alternating. I found that churning is easiest if I time the alternate pressing of each palm. Experiment and have fun. Inhale and exhale completely between sides.

Note: When "moving" the abdominal mass, the air is always completely out of the body.

Chapter 15

Where I Look
When Doing Yoga

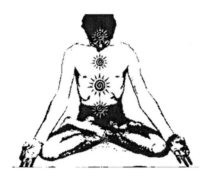

*He who is in love is wise and is becoming wiser, sees newly every
time he looks at the object beloved, drawing from it with his eyes
and his mind those virtues which it possesses.*
—RALPH WALDO EMERSON

*Look well into thyself; there is a source of strength which will
always spring up if thou wilt always look there.*
—MARCUS AURELIUS ANTONINUS

Love looks not with the eyes, but with the mind.
—WILLIAM SHAKESPEARE

In yoga, there are specific gazing points in each asana or posture.
In order to help focus the attention, each pose has a specific
place for the practitioner to gaze. It might be the tip of the nose, the
fingertips, between the eyes, the navel, off in the distance. Each
asana has a gazing point or *dristi*.

I have a confession.

As long as I am being up front about everything else regarding my yogic journey, I might as well tell you that the dristis, like the bandhas, fell into the optional category for the first two years of my practice.

All that stuff to remember! And since I was practicing at home and had no one to tell me I was a bad man or fine me $50 dollars for looking where I wasn't supposed to, I looked wherever I wanted. The mirror, at the wall, at the clock; if I did any dristi in those first two years, I assure you it was strictly accidental.

But, alas, in my quest to discover the sublime wisdom in these "suggestions" like bandhas and dristis, I eventually succumbed to observing the dristis, and I found immediately that my mind didn't wander as much.

Since most of our information is taken in visually, I understand now what a huge distraction the Wandering Eye brand of yoga I practiced those first two years was.

The best way I can illustrate the difference between Wandering Eye Yoga and a practice that incorporates dristis is by these two examples:

1. With your eyes open, take 10 deep breaths and try and still your mind. Count off each breath silently, but leave your eyes open and let them wander wherever they will in the room. Just focus on the breathing and getting to 10. Inhale for five counts and exhale for five counts. An easy way to count then is by mentally counting on the inhale: "1, 2, 3, 4, 5" and exhaling "1, 2, 3, 4, 5." That's one. Then, for the next cycle, "2, 2, 3, 4, 5" and exhaling "2, 2, 3, 4, 5." That's two. All the way up to 10.

2. Now, stare at the tip of your nose. Don't look away. Do the same breathing and counting method described above.

See what I mean?

For me, breathing (and practicing) with a focused gaze helped me slow down the train of thoughts until the thoughts came fewer and farther between and eventually slowed to a halt.

When I focused my gaze on a specific point, I was able to focus my mind.

Chapter 16

What I Eat

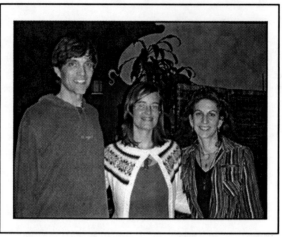

*Left to right: Me, Angela Stokes
(lost over 160 lbs. eating Raw Food) and Kathy*

Nothing will benefit human health and increase the chances for survival of life on Earth as much as the evolution to a vegetarian diet.
—ALBERT EINSTEIN

Tell me what you eat, and I will tell you what you are.
—ANTHELME BRILLAT-SAVARIN

*Why does man kill? He kills for food. And not only food:
frequently there must be a beverage.*
—WOODY ALLEN, *Without Feathers*

*Part of the secret of success in life is to eat what you like and let
the food fight it out inside.*
—MARK TWAIN

I think the reason that we are on the Planet is to experience joy.

In order to experience joy, you need to feel good. Feeling good happens when you are thinking positive thoughts. It is also a product of the company you keep, the books you read, the things you watch (or do not watch) on television, where you live, and, this is a big one, what you eat.

You are what you eat. I am what I eat.

You're okay. I'm okay.

Conscious Eating

I think food is experienced on several levels:

Decision—I'm hungry, so what do I want to put in my body? This decision can be either conscious or unconscious. Unconscious decisions may result in you eating what's cheap and/or convenient. Conscious decisions about what to eat might be more thoughtful: What food makes me feel good and is good for me, based on my experience? What food choices are the best for the Planet? What food choices support local businesses? What food choices available to me are in their natural, most organic state?

Acquisition—The process you undertake to get your food. This can be as simple as going outside and picking some herbs from a pot outside your front door or some berries growing on a bush in a field. On the other end of the spectrum, it can be as complex as driving an hour to the grocery store to buy a bunch of bananas that have traveled thousands of miles in airplanes, trucks, and finally, were stickered and arranged on a display by someone who wishes they'd never abandoned their dream of becoming a pop singer. If you are going the more complex acquisition route, consider who has handled your food? Did happy hands powered by a joyful heart handle your food? Or are you eating the energy of resentment and anger along with your soup, slammed down hurriedly on the counter by an over-worked soul who isn't thinking about what you're putting in your body for nourishment at all, but really wishes they were home hugging their children?

Preparation—Do you prepare your own food or does someone else prepare it? I think that preparing food for yourself and others is a wonderful expression of love, not a chore or a hassle. Watch someone perform the tea ceremony then watch someone put a cup of water in a microwave with a string dangling over the side of the cup with a tag on it. I promise, each tea will taste different.

Consumption—How does the food smell? How does it taste? How does it feel in your stomach?

Digestion—How do you feel a half an hour after you eat … an hour later … two hours later? The next day?

Assimilation—Does the food convert to quality energy that makes you feel good? Does it make you feel bad? Tired? Energetic?

Elimination—When your plumbing is working well, anything you eat should pass through within 24 hours. Want to test your plumbing? Eat some corn and notice how long before you see it pass out the other end. If you have it for dinner, does it appear the next morning? The next afternoon or three days later or does it go into some kind of digestive Bermuda Triangle, like Amelia Earhart, never to be heard from again?

Going Raw

People are curious about what other people eat. When people go to the grocery store, they often look at what other people are putting in their carts. Then, I have observed that they give the person the once over. I guess they want to see how the people's food choices are working out for them. Consciously or unconsciously, we are always evaluating our food choices and we are interested in what other people eat.

So, after all that, what do I eat? Christine asked me to narrate my practice, sure, but my yoga is much more than the poses that I practice. Yoga means union, connecting or re-connecting to Spirit, the part of everyone, everything and me that is underneath the forms we inhabit temporarily, that Great Unseen Energy Field that projects itself on to the big Movie Screen that all of it plays itself out upon. Therefore, my practice also includes the food I eat.

Food-wise, I have been everything …

84

I've eaten fast food, junk food and everything in between. However, about a year after starting yoga, I found that meat did not really agree with me any more.

I have experimented with just about every form of eating.

I have always eaten whatever I wanted. Someone told me that after I started doing yoga I'd eventually become a vegetarian.

Yeah, right.

I'd been a vegetarian before and even a vegan for a year. But not a serious vegetarian, just a pick-the-sausage-off-the-pizza, hold-the-baloney kind.

Serveral years ago, I was visiting some family. At dinner, out of hospitality, they offered me the biggest filet mignon on the platter. I ate it all and I remember for the next few mornings as I did yoga, I felt like an anaconda, that 12-ounce ball of meat slowly sliding along the 30-some-odd feet of plumbing searching for the light.

Go to the light! Go to the light!

That was the last piece of meat I ate.

As my yoga practice deepened, I started giving more and more thought to the food I ate.

When I met my wife Kathy, she was about three stages beyond my food evolution. She turned me on to the wonderful world of organic produce. I remember the first time I ate an organic Fuji apple.

Whoa. Nature's candy.

She gave me a bunch of books to read from what I loving refer to as The Metaphysical Library, a four-shelf collection of books in the corner of our living room that runs the gammet of subjects such as, Crystals, Reiki, Reflexology, Herbology, Self-Help, Yoga, Mysticism, and yes, Food.

All the books aside, it was watching Kathy in the kitchen that awakened me to the importance of preparing meals with love.

There's a framed picture in our kitchen that I made. It has a rainbow swirl background and bears the Sanskrit characters and English translation of one of the Upanishads: "He who gives food finds happiness."

Yes he does.

Eventually, we stopped eating dairy products and became vegan. About a year later, we started experimenting with raw food and that is where we are at now. Who knows where the rest of life will take us?

Do you know about raw food?

A lot of people who haven't really experienced raw food will, when you mention raw food, conjure in their mind the image of skinny people in Birkenstocks eating carrot sticks and organic apples, peddling their bicycles to their job at the farm co-op and back home to their off-the-grid Earth home in the commune in Oregon at the edge of the forest that they saved from clear-cutting due to a well-publicized 10-day fast during which they chained themselves naked to the trees in front of the bulldozers singing *We Shall Overcome* and *This Land is Your Land.*

(Not quite, but it is certainly something to picture, is it not?)

So what is raw food? Simply put, it is anything eaten from plant or animal sources that has not been heated to greater than 118 degrees Fahrenheit. Dry, sprout, blend, chop, grind, dehydrate, and/or soak.

Anyone who has not tried raw food, would be amazed if they tried eating raw food for 30 days.

Get some cook books out of your library. Kathy checked out every book on raw food from our local library and even bought some of the keepers.

Check out the end of this book. I've included some good books that'll help get you started.

Want some inspiration? Search www.youtube.com for "raw food" or www.rawfoodmedia.com.

Work it into your meals gradually. You can start with using organic produce and making smoothies for breakfast. There, you are 30% raw, more or less.

Add in a healthy organic green salad for lunch and some organic nuts and you're half-way there.

You might even like the way raw food makes you feel. Like us, You might even decide to go 100% raw. An easy way to tell? Your dog will stop begging for your food.

Eat raw, feel good, live long.

Chapter 17

Try Yoga for 30 Days ...
I Dare You

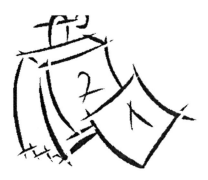

It is common sense to take a method and try it. If it fails, admit it frankly and try another. But above all, try something.
—FRANKLIN D. ROOSEVELT

What people say you cannot do, you try and find that you can.
—HENRY DAVID THOREAU

I read that about 25 million people in the United States alone say they want to try yoga every year.

I'm not sure how many of them get past the coginitive part of the decision and actually go find a class somewhere, have a friend show them a few poses, get a DVD or a book and roll out a mat and give it a whirl.

So, here's my challenge: Try yoga.

I'm not talking about doing it once and saying, "Oh, I stink at that" and throwing in the towel.

I've been at it for seven years and I still look forward to practice. David Williams has been practicing for nearly 40 years. To hear him talk about yoga, you'd think he just learned yesterday. All that enthusiasm.

How many other activities besides walking can you do your whole life?

I always tell Kathy I want to be that gnarly old man with the light still shining in his eyes when I'm 108 years old, rolling his mat out each morning to breathe deep, bend his body and feel joyful and alive.

You have read this far and I think you owe it to yourself to try yoga if you're not already practicing. Whether you go out and find a class in your area, borrow some tapes or DVD's from the library, or use another resource like a book or the internet, give yoga a try. Try it for 30 days.

I've provided a simple yoga practice here that takes no more than 15 minutes to do. Kathy and I call this practice The Minimum, meaning, if we only have a little time or a little energy, we try and at least practice what's described below. Re-read the sections on Bandhas, Breathing, Dristi and Nauli.

This simple yoga practice, The Minimum, consists of:

1. Nauli (re-read the chapter on Nauli and begin your practice with this)
2. Three Sun Salutation A's
3. Three Sun Salutation B's
4. Three Finishing Postures
5. Shavasana (corpse posture) for five minutes

Sun Salutation A
Suryanamaskar—Salutation to the Sun

Note: This book was intended to share my personal story and my yoga journey to inspire you. Most people learn yoga the quickest by watching and imitating or via the guidance of physical teacher. Second best would be a yoga tape or dvd—again a means of access to visual learning and imitation. Learning yoga from a book alone would be my last recommendation, including my book. So, if you don't have access to a physical teacher, or someone who can show you the Sun Salutations so you can follow along, do what I did: get a yoga tape. Watching someone do it will connect the dots faster in your body and mind. After you've connected some of those dots, come back to this section of the book and it is my hope that some of my words might help water an already sprouting yoga seed. I highly recommend that this book be a supplement, but that you also seek a qualified teacher. Remember my teachers: Bryan Kest's Power Yoga tapes, the Yoga With Richard Freeman Ashtanga Yoga: The Primary Series" tape, and David Williams himself, as well as others. If you've never done yoga before, just reading the practice section of this book and trying to follow along might be challenging, to say the least. I think it would be much easier to get a tape or better, experience a class and then look to this book's practice section as an additional reference.

All that said, let me say a word on Sun Salutation A.

The diagram on page 90 shows the major movements of Sun Salutation A. Unless specified otherwise in the text, you want to try to move from one position to the other in about five-second intervals. For example, if you look at the diagram, it will, with a little practice, take you about five seconds to move from the first position, standing with the hands in prayer position, to standing with the arms stretched over head, palms together, gaze on the thumbs. The only position you'll stay in for five full breaths is position number 7 (Downward Dog).

After writing this and trying to link the thumbnail diagrams to the actual description, I appreciated just how difficult it is to convey physical activity in the written word alone!

Suryanamaskar A is a foundational asana in many styles of yoga. Suryanamaskar A is a logical joining of several distinct asanas in a flow. Each asana in the flow, as well as the transitional movements between asanas, are punctuated by a series of inhales and exhales. All of these transitional movements are strung together to form a beautiful sequence that can act be a practice all by itself.

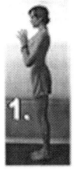

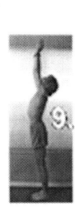

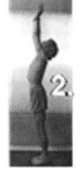

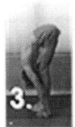

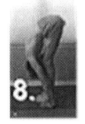

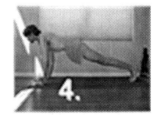

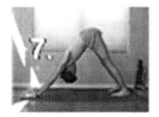

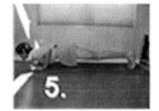

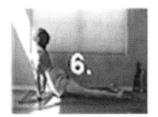

1. Standing to Forward Fold

a. From the Standing Prayer Position (*see diagram page 90, thumbnail diagram 1*), establish Maha Bandha, drop you hands to your sides and begin a long, slow inhale, turning your palms outward, fingers and thumbs spread wide.

b. Still inhaling, keep turning your palms outward until you feel your shoulder sockets rolling back and down.

c. Slowly bring your arms up overhead and before the palms touch, release Jalandhara Bandha and gently let your headdrop back slightly, while simultaneously reaching the center of your chest skyward, so that as your palms touch, your gaze settles on your thumbs (*see diagram page 90, thumbnail diagram 2*).

d. The duration of your inhale should last the length of time it takes for your palms to turn outward and the palms come together (try five slow counts).

e. Your chest remains completely lifted and open and the body should feel at its maximum length.

f. Your neck is relaxed and your throat is open.

g. Gracefully begin your exhale as you bend at the tops of your thighbones.

h. Imagine yourself from the side, folding neatly at the tops of your thighbones like a sheet of paper folding in half.

i. Your hands part and the palms open out like a book opening, like dramatically parting curtains, and you hinge forward, back straight from the tail to the crown of the head as if you are doing a swan dive.

j. Your gaze turns upward to focus between and slightly above the eyebrows, and as you fold forward, keep extending outward with the crown of your head and chest from the tail.

k. Keep pulling up the kneecaps with the thighs to help release the hamstrings.

l. 2/3rds of the way through your "dive" toward the floor, engage Jalandhara Bandha, but the Mula and Uddiyana Bandhas remain engaged.

m. There is no strain to hold the stomach in, as the extension of your chest forward and outward draws the stomach in and the waist becomes long and narrow.

n. Imagine that pull of the skin across your abdomen, as your extension between the crown of the head and the opposing movement away from the crown. The spine like a bow being drawn back by an archer, creates a hollow in the abdominal cavity—feel the area above your pubic bone draw up to your navel as it presses itself back to kiss the spine.

o. The skin on the back and shoulders flows down the back in opposition to the lift of the chest outward.

p. Your shoulders open and as your "dive" gracefully folds you in half, the top of the head extends out away from the body and down toward the feet. Just like the folding paper you are imagining, the chest points to the mat in front of your feet and the hands settle on the floor on either side of your feet, fingers together and facing forward.

q. Feel the triangle of your pelvis folding over the tops of the thighs, keep your back straight as possible, and feel the fold line at the very top of the thighbones, not the back of the waist or hamstrings at all.

r. Focus on the thigh muscles drawing up the kneecaps; the knees remain straightened, not locked.

s. Your arms extend out and down in line with and slightly behind the line of the forward moving upper body … like an exaggerated bow—as the name implies, you are bowing to the Sun.

t. Bring your fingers and hands to the floor when your fold is complete, and, if possible, keep your legs straight (*see diagram page 90, thumbnail diagram 3*). Bend your knees as much as you need to get your hands on the floor first, and begin to straighten until the chest begins to move away from the top of the thighs. Stop here! Respect your back and hamstrings and allow yourself to warm slowly.

u.   Lift your toes, curling back, and then down again to re-estab-
     lish your feet's even pressure into the mat to connect you with
     the earth.

v.   If there is strain in your back, you may need to bend your legs
     slightly, but **be happy where you are**.

w.   You may want to try just settling the palms above your knees or
     on your shins, focusing on the folded extension of the straight
     back and the length of the spine from the tail to the crown of
     the head, and the Bandhas, and not any thought or goal or
     yourself with your hands on the floor.

x.   As you gain more flexibility, the palms may move back further
     and further parallel outside the edges of the feet until the heels
     of the hands are even with the heels of the feet, but always be
     happy where you are.

y.   Shift your gaze now to the tip of the nose.

z.   The duration of the exhale should be long and steady. It begins
     from where you started with your palms touching overhead
     and ends when the lungs are emptied when you are where
     you ended up. For a guide, try to have the length of the move-
     ment and exhale last for a slow count of five.

*Smile gently and feel happy all the way through this movement.
Let the sound and texture of the breath lead and encourage the
movement of the body.*

2. Forward Fold to Looking Up

a.   Without changing the position of your legs (and moving only
     your upper body), inhale slowly and extend as far as you can
     from your tail to the crown of your head, focusing on raising
     the chest, releasing Jaladhara Bandha, and letting your head
     fall back.

b.   Let your gaze shift from the tip of the nose to the place
     between and slightly above the eyebrows.

c.   Rise up as far as you can comfortably while keeping your
     palms on the floor beside your feet. If your hands are on one of
     the alternate positions on the shins or legs, during the lift of the

chest, the shift in gaze, from the tip of the nose to the area above the eyebrows, remains the same.

d.   The duration of the inhale should be long and steady, and as in the previous movement, try and keep the sound and texture even and use as an example the same slow count of five, which helps act as an internal gauge to the duration. Eventually, the internal counting goes away, and the sound of your breath's duration has a beautiful sound, and like a musician, the durations of the inhales and exhales, the texture and sound, are the notes played along to accompany your practice.

3. Jumping or Walking Back & Lowering from Plank

a.   Exhale and walk back, one foot at a time or lightly jump both feet back into a Plank position with the arms straightened, but not locked (see diagram page 90, thumbnail diagram 4) and then slowly lower into an arms, bent push-up position with the body off the floor (see diagram page 90, thumbnail diagram 5). Imagine seeing yourself from the side—a straight line from your shoulders down along side your body to the heels.

b.   If you jumped back, work on landing lightly on the balls of your feet, feet about six to eight inches apart, landing so lightly as if your body had no weight, floating slowly onto the mat, like a feather landing soundlessly on the petal of a flower.

c.   If you are very flexible, when you jump back, shift your weight fully onto your hands, keeping your knees straightened and allow your feet to "float" back.

d.   Your arms are bent and your hands are next to your sides between your hipbones and the sides of your chest, the elbows in close to your body, and your toes curled under. Feel a slight stretch in the soles of the feet between the balls and the heels.

e.   Evenly distribute your weight on your hands and the balls of your feet.

f.   The tips of the index fingers and the thumbs gently press the earth.

g.   The back is straight and the tailbone is tucked slightly.

h.   Keep extending out from the tail out through the crown of the head and chest and feel the Mula and Uddiyana Bandhas which hold the stomach in, making a long and narrow band of strength in the waist.

i.   If you can, keep your body off the floor in a push up position. If not, that's okay, just rest your knees on the floor or let yourself all the way down onto your chest.

j.   The duration of the exhale, from jumping or walking back to the lower and hold position is long and steady and has the same slow count of five.

k.   Keep your eyes focused on the tip of your nose.

4. Rolling into Upward Dog

a.   Inhale, rolling forward over the toes, from the balls of the feet onto the tops of the feet.

b.   Gently engage the Maha Bandha, then release the Jalandhara Bandha and focus on the Mula and Uddiyana Bandhas— bringing your awareness to the perineum and the lower abdominal regions.

c.   Your weight should be evenly balanced through the tops of each foot, pressing down into the earth.

d.   Using your thigh muscles, pull up on the kneecaps, tucking your tailbone under—your legs remain straight, but your knees are not locked and your ankles relax completely, and roll outward slightly.

e.   Draw yourself up to your fullest height, imagine the opposing forces as the feet simultaneously ground and sink into the earth like the roots of a tree and the crown of the head lifts higher and higher into the sky. Imagine a space between each vertebra from the tail to your crown (see diagram page 90, thumbnail diagram 6).

f.   Keeping lifting your chest higher, until the skin on the abdomen is drawn tight from the front of the lowest ribs to the pubic bone, pressing the navel back to the spine, imagining your heart itself is lifting and opening like a flower in bloom.

g. Work the shoulder blades back, down and rise up through the crown of the head, shifting the gaze to the area up and between the eyebrows.

h. The duration of the inhale should be long and steady and as in the previous movement—try and keep the sound and texture even and use the same slow count of five, which helps act as an internal gauge to the duration from the lowered from Plank position to the Upward Facing Dog.

5. Pushing into Downward Facing Dog

a. Exhale, roll back over the tops of the toes toward the balls of your feet pushing your hips back and up toward the sky (*see diagram page 90, thumbnail diagram 7*).

b. From the side, your body forms a triangle with the apex being your tailbone, which reaches up from the tips of your index fingers, which are pressing into the mat and sinking into the earth, the weight distributed evenly across the hands with a slightly inward focus on the tips of the index fingers and thumbs.

c. Imagine that you are pulling your hips away from your fingers and your fingers away from your hips in opposite directions with the torso and spine pulled gently like a rubber band, stretching easily and lengthening by the opposing pull. Imagine a space between each vertebrae opening and releasing any accumulated waste.

d. Now imagine another line between the outer edges of the tops of your sit bones and the outer edges of your heels, which gently work themselves toward the floor. Feel happy.

e. Using your thigh muscles, pull up on the kneecaps—your legs are straight, but your knees are not locked. Roll the inner thighs inward and back to the rear.

f. Move the crown of your head down toward the floor with no strain in the back of the neck and shift your gaze toward your navel which pressing back to kiss the spine.

g. Open your chest and spread your shoulders out, back and as far from the ears as you can with no strain.

h.   Gently be aware of the Mula and Uddiyana Bandhas—bringing your attention to the perineum (cervix) and the lower abdominal regions.

i.   Your weight balances through the tops of each foot, pressing down into the earth.

j.   Keep extending out from the tail out through the top of the crown of the head and chest and feel the Mula and Uddiyana Bandhas which hold the stomach in, making a long and narrow band of strength in the waist. Concentrate on opening the chest and simultaneous pressing back the tail between the legs drawing the skin tight and long, focusing on the hollowness just above the pubic bone.

k.   Keep moving the musculature of the butt outward and apart.

l.   Imagine a gentle hand pressing your lower back flat and another set of hands of your internal teacher who stands behind you, pulling the hips gently back and up, a pair of hands circling around from behind to hold the tops of the thigh bones.

m.   Inhale and exhale now five times each. The duration of each inhale and exhale should be long and steady. Try keeping the sound and texture even and use the same slow count of five for each inhale and each exhale, which helps act as an internal gauge to the duration. Inhale, 2, 3 4, 5 ... exhale 2,3,4,5. Eventually these 5-second inhales and exhales will not require counting or conscious thought at all.

6. Jumping or Walking Up & Looking Up

a.   Begin inhaling and look up between your hands.

b.   You can walk, one foot at a time up between your hands, or

c.   Bend your knees slightly, staying on the balls of your feet, keeping your back straight, and jump both feet up between your hands with bent legs, or

d.   If you are really flexible, float up, by bending your knees slightly, staying on the balls of your feet, and push off, imagining that your tail moves into an arc up above the space between your hands, letting your weight shift over your hands as if you were coming up into a hand stand. Your legs straighten and when your tail is directly over the space between your hands, your straightened legs come back toward your torso and the feet gently settle to the floor.

e.   However your method of transport, when both feet are forward, extend as far as you can from your tail to the crown of your head, raising the chest.

f.   Let your gaze to the tip of the nose to the place between and slightly above the eyebrows.

g.   Rise up as far as you can comfortably while keeping your palms on the floor beside your feet. If your hands are on one of the alternate positions on the shins or legs, during the lift of the chest, the shift in gaze remains the same.

h.   The duration of the inhale lasts all the way through the transition from Downward Dog to the Looking Up position.

7. Folding Forward

a.   Exhale and let your chest then head drop into a Forward Fold (*see diagram page 90, thumbnail diagram 8*).

b.   The duration of the exhale lasts all the way through the transition from Looking Up to the Forward Fold.

8. Forward Fold to Arms Raised/Palms Together Position

a.   Inhale and come up, concentrating on the Mula and Uddiyana Bandhas, and think of the piece of paper being unfolded, with the fold point being the tops of the thighbones, returning to the Arms Raised Palms together position.

b.   The gaze shifts from the nose at the bottom of Forward Fold, to the point up and between the eyebrows as your reverse your swan dive back up, to the thumbs (*see diagram page 90, thumbnail diagram 9*).

c.   The duration of the

d.   inhale lasts all the way through the transition.

9. Arms Raised/Palms Together to Standing

Exhale slowly and return to Standing for the same slow count of five (return the beginning position, *page 90, thumbnail diagram 1*).

Sun Salutation B

Suryanamaskar B builds upon the foundational movements intro-
duced in Suryanamaskar A, adding two additional postures:
Utkatasana (Fierce Posture) and Virabhadrasana (Warrior Posture) A.

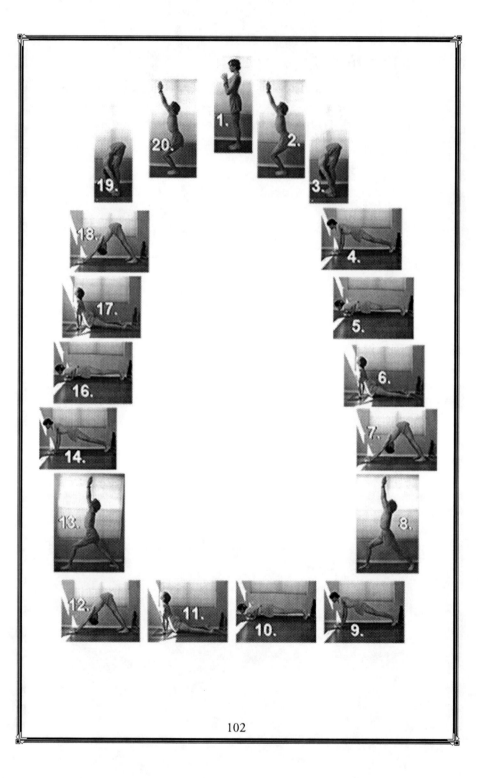

1. Standing to Utkatasana

a. From Standing, begin a long, slow inhale, turning your palms outward, and keep your fingers together.

b. Still inhaling, keep turning your palms outward until you feel your shoulder sockets rolling back and down.

c. Slowly bring your arms up overhead and while simultaneously reaching the center of your chest skyward, until your palms touch.

d. At the same time you were inhaling and bringing your hands up and together, bend your knees slightly, establish Maha Bandha, then release Jalandhara Bandha to turn your gaze up to settle on your thumbs (Utkatasana looks *like you're sitting in an invisible pointing your finger tips toward the sky with your palms together—see diagram page 100, thumbnail diagram 2*).

e. The duration of your inhale should last the length of time from Samasthitih to when the palms come together and your knees to bend (try five slow counts).

f. Your chest remains completely lifted and open and the body should feel at its maximum length.

g. Your neck is relaxed and your throat is open.

2. Utkatasana to a Forward Fold

a. Gracefully begin your exhale, and straighten your legs.

b. Your hands part and the palms open out like a book opening, like dramatically parting curtains, and you hinge forward, back straight from the tail to the crown of the head as if you are doing a swan dive.

c. Imagine yourself from the side, folding neatly at the tops of your thighbones like a sheet of paper folding in half, focusingthe "fold point" at the tops of the thighbones (see *diagram page 100, thumbnail diagram 3*).

d. Your gaze turns upward to focus between and slightly above the eyebrows, and as you fold forward, keep extending outward with the crown of your head and chest from the tail.

e. Keep pulling up the kneecaps with the thighs to help release the hamstrings.

f. The Mula and Uddiyana Bandhas remain engaged.

g. There is no strain to hold the stomach in, as the extension of your chest forward and outward draws the stomach in and the waist becomes long and narrow. Imagine that pull of the skin across your abdomen, as your extension between the crown of the head and the opposite pulling back of tailbone, which creates a hollow in the abdominal cavity, and feel the area above your pubic bone up to your navel as it presses itself back to kiss the spine.

h. The skin on the back and shoulders flows down the back in opposition to the lift of the chest outward.

i. Your shoulders open and as your "dive" gracefully folds you in half, the top of the head extends out away from the body and down toward the feet. Just like the folding paper you are imagining, the chest points to the mat in front of your feet and the hands settle on the floor on either side of your feet, fingers together and facing forward.

j. Feel the triangle of your pelvis folding over the tops of the thighs, keep your back straight as possible, and feel the fold line at the very top of the thighbones, not the back of the waist or hamstrings at all.

k. Focus on the thigh muscles drawing up the kneecaps, with the knees straightened, not locked.

l. About 2/3rds of the way into your dive re-engage the Maha Bandha, by tucking your chin in to Jalandhara Bandha, and, since you're still engaging the Mula and Uddiyana Bandhas, you are now engaging the Maha Bandha (the "Great Lock" or simultaneous engagement of the Mula, Uddiyana & Jalandhara Bandhas).

m. Turn your gaze to your nose.

n. Your arms extend out to the sides and down in line with and slightly behind the line of the forward moving upper body.

o. Bring your fingers and hands to the floor when your fold is complete, and, if possible, keep your legs straight.

p. Lift your toes, curling back, and then down again to re-establish the even pressure of your feet into the mat to connect you with the earth.

q. If there is strain in your back, you may need to bend your legs slightly, but be happy where you are.

r. You may want to try just settling the palms above your knees or on your shins, focusing on the folded extension of the straight back and the length of the spine from the tail to the crown of the head, and the Bandhas, and not any thought or goal or yourself with your hands on the floor.

s. As you gain more flexibility, the palms may move back further and further parallel outside the edges of the feet until the finger tips are even with the heels, but always be happy where you are.

t. The duration of the exhale should be long and steady. It begins from where you started with your palms touching overhead and ends when the lungs empty when you are where you ended up, and for a guide, try to have the length of the movement and exhale last for a slow count of five.

u. Smile gently and feel happy all the way through this movement. Let the sound and texture of the breath lead and encourage the movement of the body.

3. Forward Fold to Looking Up

a. Without changing the position of your legs, and moving only your upper body—inhale slowly and extend as far as you can from the tail to the crown of the head, focusing on raising the chest.

b. Let your gaze shift from the tip of the nose to the place between and slightly above the eyebrows.

c. Rise up as far as you can comfortably while keeping your fingertips on the floor beside your feet. If your hands are on one of the alternate positions on the shins or legs, during the lift of the chest, the shift in gaze remains the same.

d. The duration of the inhale should be long and steady. As in the previous movement, try keeping the sound and texture even and use as an example the same slow count of five, which helps act as an internal gauge to the duration. Eventually, the internal counting goes away, and the sound of your breath's duration has a beautiful sound, like a flute, and like a musician, the durations of the inhales and exhales, the texture and sound, are the notes played along to accompany your practice.

4. Jumping or Walking Back to Chatvari

a. Exhale and walk back, one foot at a time or lightly jump both feet back into a Plank position (see diagram page 100, thumbnail diagram 3). Keep the arms straightened but not locked and lower into an arms-bent, push-up position with the body off the floor (Chatvari), and imagine seeing yourself from the side—a straight line from your shoulders down along side your body to the heels (see diagram page 100, thumbnail diagram 4).

b. If you jumped back, work on landing lightly on the balls of your feet, feet about six to eight inches apart, landing so lightly as if your body had no weight, floating slowly onto the mat, like a feather landing soundlessly on the petal of a flower.

c. If you are very flexible, when you jump back, shift your weight fully onto your hands, keeping your knees straightened and allow your feet to "float" back.

d. Your arms are bent and your hands are next to your sides between your hipbones and the sides of your chest, the elbows in close to your body, and your toes curled under. Feel a slight stretch in the soles of the feet between the balls and the heels.

e. Evenly distribute your weight on your hands and the balls of your feet.

f. The tips of the index fingers and the thumbs gently press the earth.

g.	The back is straight and the tailbone tucks slightly.

h.	Keep extending out from the tail out through the crown of the head and chest and feel the Mula and Uddiyana Bandhas which hold the stomach in, making a long and narrow band of strength in the waist.

i.	If you can, keep your body off the floor in a push up position. If not, that's okay, just rest your knees on the floor or let yourself all the way down onto your chest.

j.	The duration of the exhale, from jumping or walking back to the lower and hold position is long and steady and has the same slow count of five.

k.	Keep your eyes focused on the tip of your nose.

5. Chatvari to Upward Facing Dog

a.	Inhale, rolling forward over the toes, from the balls of the feet onto the tops of your feet.

b.	Gently engage the Maha Bandha.

c.	Your weight should be evenly balanced through the tops of each foot, pressing down into the earth.

d.	Using your thigh muscles, pull up on the kneecaps, tucking your tailbone under—your legs remain straight, but your knees are not locked.

e.	Draw yourself up to your fullest height, imagine the opposing forces as the feet simultaneously ground and sink into the earth like the roots of a tree and the crown of the head lifts higher and higher into the sky. Imagine a space between each vertebra from the tail to your crown (see *diagram page 100, thumbnail diagram 6*).

f.	Keeping lifting your chest higher, until the skin on the abdomen is drawn tight from the front of the lowest ribs to the pubic bone, pressing the navel back to the spine, imagining your heart itself is lifting and opening like a flower in bloom.

g.	Work the shoulder blades back and down, pushing up through the crown of the head, shifting the gaze to the area up and between the eyebrows, letting the neck gently drop back.

h. The duration of the inhale should be long and steady and as in the previous movement—try and keep the sound and texture even and use the same slow count of five, which helps act as an internal gauge to the duration from the lowered from Plank position to the Upward Facing Dog.

6. Upward Facing Dog to Downward Dog & Into Right Foot Forward Virabhadrasana A

a. Begin your exhale, rolling back over the tops of the toes toward the balls of your feet, pushing your hips back and up (*see diagram page 100, thumbnail diagram 7*).

b. From the side, your body forms a triangle with the apex being your tailbone, which reaches up from the tips of your index fingers, which are pressing into the mat and sinking into the earth. Your weight is distributed evenly across the hands with a slightly inward focus on the tips of the index fingers and thumbs.

c. Imagine that you are pulling your hips away from your fingers and your fingers away from your hips in opposite directions with the torso and spine pulled gently like a rubber band, stretching easily and lengthening by the opposing pull. Imagine a space between each vertebrae opening and releasing any accumulated waste.

d. Now imagine another line between the outer edges of the tops of your sit bones and the outer edges of your heels, which gently work themselves toward the floor. If they never reach the floor, be happy.

e. Using your thigh muscles, pull up on the kneecaps—your legs remain straight, but your knees are not locked. Roll the inner thighs inward and back to the rear of your legs.

f. Move the crown of your head down toward the floor with no strain in the back of the neck and shift your gaze toward your navel.

g. Open your chest and spread your shoulders out, back and as far from the ears as you can with no strain.

h. Gently engage Maha Banda.

i. Your weight should be evenly balanced through the tops of each foot, pressing down into the earth.

j. Keep extending out from the tail out through the crown of the head. Expand the chest and feel the Mula and Uddiyana Bandhas, which hold the stomach in, making a long and narrow band of strength in the waist. This opening of the chest and simultaneous pressing back of the tail between the legs drawing the skin tight and long, focusing on the hollowness just above the pubic bone.

k. Keep moving the musculature of the butt outward and apart.

l. Imagine a gentle hand pressing your lower back flat and another set of hands of your internal teacher who stands behind you, pulling the hips gently back and up, their fingers circling around from behind to hold the tops of the thigh bones.

m. Still exhaling, from the Downward Dog, step your right foot forward between your hands, while simultaneously shifting your left foot about 45-degrees, with the middle of the left foot perpendicular with the heel of the right foot (see *diagram page 100, thumbnail diagram 8*).

n. Focus on your feet, pressing the outer edge of the left foot evenly into the earth from your smallest toe along and back to the heel. Press the inner edge of the right foot into the earth and down … you can even lift and curl your toes, and drop to emphasize and join the feet in the "gripping" of the earth.

o. Your right knee moves out over the top of the right ankle to form and 90-degree angle with the leg, so the bottom of the thigh forms a parallel line with the earth.

p. Engage the thigh muscles of the left leg, and pull up on the kneecap.

q. The transition from the Downward Dog to this point, right knee bent, left leg straight, both palms on the floor is accomplished to accompany the sound of one long smooth exhale.

r. Now begin to inhale.

s. Engage the Maha Bandha as you bring your torso up and your palms turn up to touch, like a mini Utkatasana.

t. Just before your palms touch, you've left the Jalandhara Bandha to focus the gaze on the thumbs, allowing the neck to drop gently back.

u. The duration of the inhale lasts from the moment the feet are set and the hands begin to rise until the gaze has settled on the thumbs.

7. Virabhadrasana A Back to Chatvari

Exhaling, return to sweep both arms down and return to the push up position and then lower to Chatvari (see *diagram page 100, thumbnail diagram 9 and 10*).

8. Chatvari to Upward Dog

Inhaling, move into Upward Dog (see *diagram page 100, thumbnail diagram 11*).

9. Upward Dog to Left Foot Forward Virabhadrasana A

a. Begin your exhale and move smoothly into Downward Dog.

b. Exhale and push your hips back into Down Dog momentarily (see *diagram page 100, thumbnail diagram 12*) and while still exhaling, move into left foot forward Virabhadrasana A, switching to the inhale once your feet are set and your hands begin the ascent to the palms together position, concluding the inhale when the gaze has settled on the thumbs (see *diagram page 100, thumbnail diagram 13*).

10. Left Foot Forward Virabhadrasana A to Chatvari

Exhaling, return to sweep both arms down and return to the push up position and then lower to Chatvari (see *diagram page 100, thumbnail diagram 14 and 16—yes I know, "Where's 15?" I saw this after I'd already sent the final plates off to the publisher—*).

11. Chatvari to Upward Dog
Inhaling, move into Upward Dog (*see diagram page 100, thumbnail diagram 17*).

12. Upward Dog into Downward Dog
Exhaling, move into Downward Dog and enjoy five rounds of deep breaths, concentrating on keep the Maha Bandha and listening to the equal length of both the inhales and exhales (*see diagram page 100, thumbnail diagram 18*).

13. Downward Dog to Jumping or Walking Forward and Looking Up
a. After the last exhale in Downward Dog, begin inhaling and look up between your hands.
b. You can walk, one foot at a time up between your hands, or
c. Bend your knees slightly, staying on the balls of your feet, keeping your back straight, and jump both feet up between your hands with bent legs, or
d. If you are really flexible, float up, by bending your knees slightly, staying on the balls of your feet, and push off, imagining that your tail moves into an arc up above the space between your hands, letting your weight shift over your hands as if you were coming up into a hand stand. Your legs straighten and when your tail is directly over the space between your hands, your straightened legs come back toward your torso and the feet gently settle to the floor.
e. However your method of transportation, when both feet are forward, extend as far as you can from your tail to the crown of your head, raising the chest.
f. Let your gaze to the tip of the nose to the place between and slightly above the eyebrows.
g. Rise up as far as you can comfortably while keeping your fingertips on the floor beside your feet. If your hands are on one of the alternate positions on the shins or legs, during the lift of the chest, the shift in gaze remains the same.

h.   The duration of the inhale lasts all the way through the transition from Downward Dog to the Looking Up position.

14. Folding Forward

a.   Exhale and let your chest then head drop into a Forward Fold (*see diagram page 100, thumbnail diagram 19*).

b.   Two-thirds of the way into the Forward Fold, engaging the Maha Bandha and shift the gaze to the nose.

c.   The duration of the exhale lasts all the way through the transition from Looking Up to the end of the Forward Fold.

15. Returning to Utkatasana from the Forward Fold

a.   Inhale and come up, concentrating on the Maha Bandha, and think of the piece of paper being unfolded, the fold point being the tops of the thighbones, returning to Utkatasana (*see diagram page 100, thumbnail diagram 20*).

b.   The gaze shifts from the nose at the bottom of Forward Fold, to the point up and between the eyebrows as your reverse your swan dive back up, to the thumbs.

c.   The duration of the inhale lasts all the way through the transition.

16. Returning to Standing from Utkatasana

a.   Exhale slowly and return to Standing for the same slow count of five.

Finishing Postures

After you've done your Sun Salutations (A&B) you can begin the three finishing postures and then Savasana.

Baddha Padmasana

Baddha Padmasana—bound lotus posture

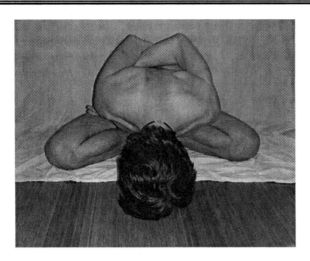

Baddha Padmasana is the sister pose to the Pindasana, revisiting the Lotus and the paradox of "binding." A common adjustment in this pose is for a teacher to gently press *forward* (not down) on the back of the student. Feel those invisible hands *gently* pressing you forward, keeping your inner eye on the bend occurring at the tops of the thighbones with no strain in the lower back. What do the heels "find" in the Lotus as they press in the lower belly and across the top of each opposite thigh? How does moving the shoulder blades out and down change the depth of the forward bend?

1. From a seated, exhale and fold the legs into the lotus or an easy cross-legged posture.
2. Engage Maha Bandha, inhale and reach the left hand behind the back and grasp the left big toe. (Note: This took me two years to do! In the beginning, I interlaced my fingers behind me, straightened my arms and slowly brought my arms over head. Take your time … you've got your whole life ahead of you.)
3. Reach the right hand behind the back and grasp the right big toe.
4. Roll the shoulders back as if to touch the shoulder blades.

5. Lift and widen the chest, release Jalandhara Bandha and let the head fall back. Inhale and look to the area above and between the eyebrows drawing up as "tall" as possible.
6. Exhale and come forward and try and touch the chin to the floor.
7. Begin a cycle of 30 breaths.
8. After the last breath, inhale, re-engaging the Jalandhara Bandha while coming back up with the gaze on the nose.

You will move into Padmasana from here.

Padmasana

Padmasana—lotus posture

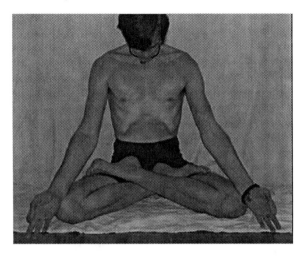

Padmasana is the Guru of all asanas.

1. From the last position of Baddha Padmasana, exhale and release your grips on the toes.
2. Engage Maha Bandha, inhale and straighten the arms, placing the backs of the hands on the knees.
3. Lightly touch the index fingers and thumbs of each hand, splaying the three remaining fingers of each hand, and rolling the wrists outward.
4. Gaze at the nose.
5. Begin a cycle of 30 breaths.

You will move into Tolasana from here.

Tolasana
Tolasana—scale posture

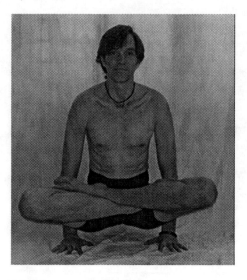

Tolasana is the lifted version of Padmasana.

1. From the last position of Padmasana, exhale and place the hands, palms down outside the hips.
2. Rolling on the sit bones, draw the lotus legs off the floor and place the palms under the thighs with the fingers splayed.
3. Inhale and engage Maha Bandha, release Jalandhara Bandha and press the buttocks off the floor and lift the lotus legs.
4. The knees are about six inches higher than the bottom of the buttocks.
5. Gaze at the nose.
6. Use the Uddiyana and Mula Bandha to assist with the lift.
7. Breath in and out strongly, working up to 108 cycles. Force the breath out your nostrils in a sudden burst each time and take a short inhale. Your breath should sound like an old-fashioned locomotive.

8. After the last breath, lower, unfold the legs.

You will move into Shavasana from here.

Shavasana

Shavasana—corpse posture

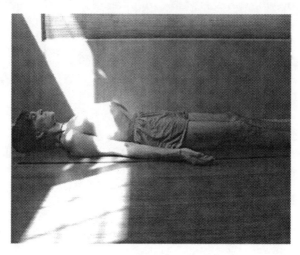

Shavasana is the final posture of the Primary Series and a deeply meditative pose. More than any other pose, Shavasana is what draws me back to my yoga practice each day.

1. Lay on your back, arms at your side, feet apart and relax and slowly roll the palms up to the sky.
2. The feet flop to either side.
3. Imagine your whole body slowly melting into the ground.

Personally, if I can, I like to cover myself with a Mexican falsa blanket to keep my body heat in as long as possible. Additionally, to help me relax, I put an eye pillow over my eyes.

Here's some things to consider when doing Shavasana:

> Where do you feel tension? Is it your hips? Is it your shoulders, your arms, your waist, lower back, hamstrings, ankles, or neck? Welcome those discoveries of tightness with a mother's compassion! Imagine there is a part of

you that has *witnessed* all your hurts, sufferings and fearful reactions (but *not* shared or felt them) since you were a child.

Acknowledge the tension is there and each time you breathe, *feel* the tension releasing; and let it go. Imagine the tension is released from the body like a liquid; and let this liquid release and disappear into the earth.

When your body is peaceful and still, imagine watching the goodness and joy of the universe entering the body through the tips of the toes, the soles of the feet. Imagine that this goodness and joy are a cool white blue light, like a tornado of love that you have summoned with the intention of receiving to nourish and fill the body. Imagine watching this love swirling and funneling from the universe and down in to your toes. Once it reaches your toes, imagine through some magical alchemy, it becomes a warm white blue liquid, traveling up the length of the legs, entering the spine, moving gently up the length of the spine, like a healing sap rising inside the stem of a flower, nourishing and healing each area of the spine.

Feel this healing love at the tail of the spine, below the navel, at the stomach, the heart, the throat, and feel yourself smiling as it passes through the roof of your mouth, above the eyebrows, opening into a beautiful blossom out the top of the crown of the head.

Lie in this position for at least five minutes. When you are finished, gently stretch the arms over your head and stiffen your legs, pointing the toes as you inhale.

Hold and exhale.

Inhale, engage Maha Bandha and draw the knees up to the chest, hugging your legs gently.

Exhale and slowly sit up and notice how good you feel. Tell your self the peace and tranquility you feel will last for the rest of the day. At any time during the day you feel you've "forgotten," remember the bliss feeling and tell yourself you're feeling it now.

Feel Good

Be happy that today you have ventured boldly into this internal world of discovery and released a powerful "current" of positive energy, healing force, prana, whatever you want to call it. This current of energy has the power to heal not only you, but it is *felt by others, too.*

This energy you feel can *heal* you and everyone you meet today.

Joy or love is like electricity, and you are like a light bulb. You can feel this love all day each time you choose positive thoughts. Today, with your positive thoughts, you will give off *light* and feel the *warmth* when love flows in you and th*rough* you.

Other people will be attracted to your light.

By choosing your thoughts of love, you choose to flip the switch that allows the current to flow. Your light bulb warms and glows brightly.

You begin to see that this electricity is everywhere, not just inside you, but also waiting inside everyone.

You see that everyone is a light bulb.

Some light bulbs need help before they can glow.

If you send enough love, through your positive thoughts, feelings and actions, know that you can encourage others to flip their switches, too.

Feel good and light your world with love.

Chapter 18

You Really Are
a Good Writer

I am a good writer

David Williams, I know someone else who attended your seminar wrote the article I read on Yoga Journal's website, but he was just "prettying" up or using his learned and practiced "skills" as a writer to capture and preserve in written format your teaching during a seminar.

As long as it's posted on yoga Journal's site, people have the potential to learn from David Williams for centuries.

(Note to Yoga Journal: Leave David Williams' article posted for downloading for centuries!)

David, even if no one has ever watered your writing seed, please know that you have one.

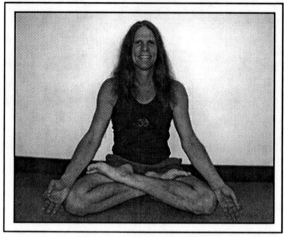

David Williams, Senior Ashtanga Yoga Instructor

Writing is just talking, or in your case, teaching on paper. David and anyone who is reading:

If I could be so presumptuous, I would love it if you felt like narrating your practice.

What thoughts did you have after you read that? Were they negative or positive?

I would like to take a moment to *overemphasize* the importance of written communication.

Are you reading this and have said these words in your head or aloud, "I wish I could write?"

How many of you have read *Autobiography of a Yogi, Light on Yoga, Moola Bandha: The Master Key* or any other number of inspiring books?

Did these books help you? If so, be glad that each of these people's writing seed was watered.

Have you ever had the experience when talking of having *just the right words come out of your mouth*?

Writing is just talking on paper.

If you are a teacher, have a desire to become a teacher, or you have something you want to say, please water your own writing seed.

Someone told me once, "You're *really* a good writer and smart!"

Back in fourth grade, someone else could have read my essay and said, "This sucks," and you might not be reading this.

Let me be your Mrs. Winings.

It's the least I can do. You see, I can never repay her or anyone else who was kind enough to encourage me until I became strong enough to encourage myself.

Mrs. Winings' greatness was in her ability to instill beliefs in a 10-year old boy who didn't believe in himself.

Even if one of you **believes** you really are a good writer after reading this and your written words help someone, I can feel I at least did my best to **encourage others**, just as I was encouraged.

Maybe *more than one* of you will **believe you really are a good writer**.

Whoever you are, "I'm afraid that novel inside you will have to come out."

Know that my book sat waiting inside me for over 30 years.

Nevertheless, for over 30 years, I believed I was a writer and I practiced writing.

I wore down the writing dendrite path.

"Practice and all is coming," as Pattabhi Jois said.

Words have the power to reach so many more people when written down and shared.

All that stands between you and becoming a writer or anything else you want to be is your desire to learn, words of encouragement and practice.

Then it is simply wearing down a dendrite path.

When you read the descriptions of the asanas, my narration of my practice, all you are reading is *my* dendrites. I have tried my best to look at all those breadcrumbs in my brain and attach words to those physical instructions, hoping that someone else would benefit from reading them.

Christine's words of encouragement created a belief in me that others could benefit from reading my dendrites. Once you get to the Practice part of this book that is all you are reading, my attempt to put words around the dendrites.

There *are* physical and time limitations on how many people can learn from you personally.

There *are no* physical or time limitations on how many people can read your written words.

Thank you for reading mine.

Aloha,

Danny Living

I Recommend ...

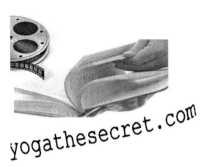

yogathesecret.com

David Williams Workshops

I think David Williams is a highly gifted teacher grounded in his experience, practical wisdom and commitment to teaching a safe, life-long yoga practice that any *body* can benefit from.

Do yourself a favor: Visit David's website at: www.ashtangayogi.com and look at his current schedule (www.ashtangayogi.com/HTML/workshops.html). You will love his workshops. They are worth every penny. Wait until you hear his Adventures in Yoga. As he says, "Yoga is for liberation! I'm not holding anything out for the next workshop!"

Tell him that you read Danny's book and you wanted to meet and experience him yourself. Introduce yourself and say, "A-lo-ha!"

Books

- Buddhananda, Swami. *Moola Bandha: The Master* Key. Munger, Bihar, India: Yoga Publicationsns Trust, 1998.
- Rampuri. *Baba: Autobiography of a Blue-Eyed Yogi.* Harmony/Bell Tower, 2005.
- Porter, Eleanor H. *Pollyanna*. Boston, The Page Company Publishers, 1913.

- Conwell, Russell H. *Acres of Diamonds*. New York: Harper & Brothers Publishers, 1915
- Patanjali. *The Yoga Sutras of Patanjali*
- Das, Ram. *Be Here Now*. Lama Foundation, 1971.
- Swenson, David. *Ashtanga Yoga: The Practice Manual: An Illustrated Guide to Personal Practice*. Ashtanga Yoga Productions, 1999.
- The Boutenko Family. *Raw Family, A True Story of Awakening*. Raw Family Publishing, 2000.
- Smith, Jeffrey. *Seeds of Deception*. Yes Books, 2003.
- Nestle, Marion. *What to Eat*. North Point Press, 2006.
- Burroughs, Stanley. *The Master Cleanse*. Burroughs Books, 1976.
- Redfield, James. *The Celestine Prophecy*. Grand Central Publishing, 1995.
- Vitale, Joe. *The Attractor Factor*. John Wiley & Sons, 2005.
- Amsden, Matt. *RAWvolution: Gourmet Living Cuisine*. New York: Regan Books, 2006.

Instructional Media
- Ashtanga Yoga with Richard Freeman: Primary Series
- Bryan Kest Power Yoga Complete Collection

DVDs
- *The Future of Food*
- *Ram Das: Fierce Grace*
- *Best Boy*
- *What the Bleep Do We Know!?*

Internet
Yoga
www.yogathesecret.com my website
www.ashtangayogi.com David Williams' website
www.ashtanga.com lots of information on Ashtanga Yoga
www.ashtanga.net David Swenson's website

Raw Food
www.borrowedearth.org Kathy Living's website
www.rawreform.com Angela Stokes
www.rawfoodmedia.com raw foodists, downloadable videos

Yoga: The Secret

What you think matters

Whether you currently practice yoga or you are interested in trying yoga, this book has something for you.

Yoga has been around for thousands of years, and according to the Yoga in America study sponsored by *Yoga Journal* magazine:

- Americans spend $2.95 billion annually on yoga classes and products
- 16.5 million U.S. adults practice yoga
- **25 million people say they intend to try yoga within the next 12 months**

While there are other books on yoga on the market, what makes this one different is that it uses the principles of the **Law of Attraction** for developing, maintaining and maximizing the benefits of yoga.

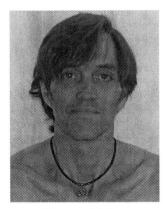

Danny Living

Danny Living is a devoted yogi and a genuinely nice, aware, and sensitive person. He has practiced yoga for many years and has great insight into what yoga is all about. I have posted "The Chemistry of Yoga" chapter from this book on my website under the Articles *section. I think that it is brilliant. I heartily recommend, Danny's book,* Yoga: The Secret, *and anything else that he may write.*

—**DAVID WILLIAMS**, Senior Ashtanga Yoga Instructor
www.ashtangayogi.com

978-0-595-44820-3
0-595-44820-8

Printed in the United States
90889LV00005B/130-168/A